Seeing Beyond Blindness

a volume in
Critical Concerns in Blindness

Series Editor:
Ronald J. Ferguson, *Louisiana Tech University*

Critical Concerns in Blindness

Ronald J. Ferguson, Series Editor

Making It Work: Educating the Blind/Visually Impaired Student in the Regular School (2005)
edited by Carol Castellano

Education and Rehabilitation for Empowerment (2005)
edited by C. Edwin Vaughan and James H. Omvig

The Blindness Revolution: Jernigan in His Own Words (2005)
edited by James H. Omvig

Seeing Beyond Blindness

by

Shelley Kinash
University of Calgary

INFORMATION AGE PUBLISHING

Greenwich, Connecticut • www.infoagepub.com

Library of Congress Cataloging-in-Publication Data

Kinash, Shelley.
Seeing beyond blindness / by Shelley Kinash.
p. cm. -- (Critical concerns in blindness)
Includes bibliographical references.
ISBN-13: 978-1-59311-521-0 (pbk.)
ISBN-13: 978-1-59311-522-7 (hardcover)
1. Blindness. 2. Blind--Research. 3. Blind--Education. 4. Computer-assisted instruction. 5. Computers and people with disabilities. I. Title. II. Series.
HV1593.K48 2006
362.4'1--dc22

200601458

ISBN 13: 978-1-59311-521-0 (pbk.)
978-1-59311-522-7 (hardcover)
ISBN 10: 1-59311-521-0 (pbk.)
1-59311-522-9 (hardcover)

Printed in the United States of America

Dedication

To Olga, Ernest, Milt, Elaine, Erich and Hadel Spitzer
and Stan, Kirsten and Josh Kinash
... for showing me what it means to be blind and what it means to see love.

CONTENTS

...

Critical Concerns in Blindness Series

A Project of the

Professional Development and Research Institute on Blindness

The Professional Development and Research Institute on Blindness was established by the Louisiana Center for the Blind in 1999 and became a center at Louisiana Tech University in October 2001. The purpose of the Institute on Blindness is to provide leadership in creating programs and conducting research that recognizes the socially constructed assumptions underpinning the current structure of the blindness system and research being done on blindness. As a result, the Institute on Blindness provides alternative programs and research that expands the boundaries of the blindness field. Currently the Institute on Blindness offers two graduate programs—orientation and mobility and teachers of blind students (often referred to as teachers of the visually impaired).

The mission of the institute is to advance the blindness field by providing the blind and professionals serving the blind with innovative programs and conducting meaningful research that will empower blind people to live independent and productive lives.

Books in the series

Making It Work: Educating the Blind/Visually Impaired Student in the Regular School (2005)
By Carol Castellano

Education and Rehabilitation for Empowerment (2005)
by C. Edwin Vaughan & James H. Omvig

The Blindness Revolution: Jernigan in His Own Words (2005)
by James H. Omvig

PREFACE

I wonder whether you are reading these words in Braille or print, or listening to them on tape or Daisy or some other digitized version. I wonder whether you have read the entire book and are only now flipping back to the preface to see what extra words I thought to tag on here, or whether you are a linear reader who starts at the beginning and reads word-for-word to the end. I wonder whether you have purchased the book, are reading the preface contemplating whether to spend your hard-earned cash, borrowing a friend's copy, whether you are at a library, and whether this version is dog-eared or fresh and crisp. I wonder what year it is now and whether my examples are still current and relevant or whether the technologies I describe herein are now historic.

It is a strange conversation between a writer and a reader. At the point at which the publisher and I decide upon fixing these words into print or some other published format, I release control of the reciprocity of the conversation and the interlocuters become you the reader and the ideas on the page. This is quite a responsibility, but an exciting prospect. Fixing the words into atoms is like striking a pose. Yet, for you the reader, the text is like the unsuspecting object of an admirer rather than a paid posed model in a drawing class. Without warning, the discourse shifts. Sometimes subtly, sometimes abruptly you change too. I remember an anonymous poster that read, "when you re-read a classic, it is not that you find something in it that you did not notice before, but that you are who you were not before." The relationship between the reader and the text is like the symbolism of art. It does not really matter what the poet or painter intends or sees when he produces an esoteric and expressive art-form. If it speaks to you, if you emotionally engage with it, if it symbolizes something to you, then it matters. I invite you into a conversation with my research, thoughts and ideas, and I hope that the captured words release your own contemplations.

Inside this book are reflections on the nature of vision and blindness. Further, there are explorations of interpretive research, and presentations of some seminal and contemporary publications in the field of blindness. The other major fodder for conversation with you the reader is an elaborated example of empirical research entitled *Blind Online Learners*. Each element of this inquiry is explicitly reflected upon as an example of interpretive research.

This book is intended for four intersecting groups of readers. If you are a philosopher, closet or sanctioned, then you cannot ponder the nature of being without due consideration for vision, and cannot contemplate the role of seeing in our lives without listening to the stories of those who are blind. The tales within this text are particularly contemporaneous because they are contextualized by the cyber-phenomena of online learning. This segues to the second group of readers, as the described empirical research was originally intended to bring greater depth and breadth of understanding to the field of educational technology, particularly as it intersects with disability studies. There is a paucity of published literature that has inquired into disabled online learners, and this research study responds to that call. Third, this book may be used as a textbook on approaches to interpretive empirical research. It is as close as one may come to a recipe, walking students through a specific example. Because it is situated in actual empirical research, the intention was that it avoid the trap of being prescriptive or formulaic. Finally, the text is intended for readers interested in the field of blindness. The text reviews some of the seminal and contemporary research on blindness, and then presents an elaborated example of what we can and should expect to emerge in the knowledge production industry, changing what it means to be blind.

Each of the participants' stories were constructed in the meeting of the horizons of experience and perceptions of each informant and the researcher. It is posited that the stories would have differed in their depiction with another researcher. The researcher is not a neutral party. I brought values, ideas, and expectations based on what I have read and experienced within a cultural context. As such, my autobiography and particularly how I came to the research needs to be shared.

Both my introduction to personal computers and my first personal experience of blindness transpired in the pivotal teen years. Visits to my Dad's office and more specifically to the room that housed the giant computer and its multicolored punch cards ignited a passion in my brother. Multiple iterations of the personal computer came to find its rightful place in our home. While our friends played on the Atari game system, my brother programmed our Atari computer. He taught me some "basic" and we demonstrated the Vic20 and the Commodore64 at the Zellers department store. I never got much past making my name fill the screen and then scroll vertically. He went on to bring home newer and "brighter" computers, earned through winning computer competitions. He tried to convince me to use word processing software to produce my junior high school papers, but after the computer "ate" them a couple times, I went back to paper and pen. My brother now lives in the Silicon Valley and manipulates operating systems and directs innovative technical design projects.

Within that same teen period, we were paid a visit by my Dad's Tante Hadel and Onkel Erich from Germany, and a year or so later, my family and I returned the visit to Germany. Upon finishing high school I returned. I spent 6 months back-packing through Europe, spending a month in their home. Onkel Erich and I were particularly taken with one another. To this day, he continues to call me his Canadian daughter. He has a hearty laugh and makes many jokes to inspire it. He takes pride in fitness—swimming many laps each morning. And he is blind.

Each spring from my 14th year onward I would look for a summer job to fill my time and purse. One summer I was tired of the regular choices of fast food and clothing retail, and I could no longer ride on the coat-tails of my brother as computer education had moved well-beyond my knowledge of Basic. I applied at the Baker Centre—Calgary's local institution for people with developmental disabilities. I was hired to work in the adult residence as an institutional aide. For my first day initiation, my new colleagues lined the men up down the hall (naked) and I bathed them. It was despicable and a humiliating experience for me and for the men. Still I returned the next summer as well. Then, I completed a bachelor's degree in English literature and communications studies. Upon graduation I was hired as coordinator of a community job placement program for adults with developmental disabilities. I assumed a number of positions all in the interests of promoting socially valued roles and meaningful relationships with people with disabling conditions. I completed my master's degree in community rehabilitation and spent 11 years as faculty in Community Rehabilitation And Disability Studies (CRDS) at the University of Calgary in Canada.

In the process, I married a wonderful man and gave birth to two children. Upon returning from my second maternity leave, my director and I decided that I would coordinate our online learning initiatives. At the same time I began my doctoral studies in educational technology.

CRDS, a program within the faculty of education at the University of Calgary, has been offering distance education since its inception over 20 years ago. In 1995 we launched our online courses with three quarter-courses dedicated to understanding anatomy, physiology, and health foundations of disabling conditions across the life span. By 2003, we offered 25 online courses. The program can be considered a case study in online learning management. We began by hiring one of our own graduate students for coordination of instructional design and course delivery. The single position quickly evolved into a team, including technicians to design and administer specially designed interfaces including online bulletin boards and chat rooms, and to produce educational digital videos. We then supported the team to form a company. We became their main contracting source. Other contracts came from within the faculty of education at large and from corporate Calgary.

Our decision, in 2000, to discontinue contracting the company we had initiated was not taken lightly. The primary reason was that the University of Calgary had been dedicating efforts to establish unified systems and resources for the development and delivery of online courses across faculties and programs. A site license was now carried for the learning moderation system—WebCT, followed by a transition to Blackboard. University-wide systems and procedures handled administrative issues such as course population and password assignment. The Learning Commons unit offered consultation with instructional developers, numerous faculty development courses and an intensive spring working symposium.

I became increasingly interested in inquiry into what it is like to be an online learner, and how postsecondary institutions are beginning to adopt a student-centered approach. I wrote a proposal to use the Community Rehabilitation and Disability Studies students in a qualitative case study.

In June 2002 I attended the Second Annual Second City Conference on Disability Studies and Education in Chicago. The night before the conference began I sat reading a stack of journal articles and came across one by Kim-Rupnow, Dowrick, and Burke (2001). Their search of journal article indexes revealed a total of eight articles about disabled postsecondary students. I was astounded. The keynote address on the opening evening of the conference steeled my resolve to move beyond postsecondary learners studying disability, to the disabled postsecondary students themselves. As the disability rights slogan and that keynote address so aptly proclaim—"nothing about us without us."

On the final day of the conference, I had lunch with Dr. Ron Ferguson, author of the ground-breaking book, *We Know Who We Are*, and who was at that time Senior Research Fellow for the Professional Development and Research Institute on Blindness (Institute on Blindness) at Louisiana Tech University. We discussed the applicability of the research to the blind. It made sense to begin an inquiry with blind learners given that blind postsecondary students were among the leaders of social justice movements at institutions such as Bęrkeley (Shapiro, 1993). In addition, I had often thought about the visual nature of the computer interface. How did blind users fare? I submitted a new research proposal and support was confirmed on August 1, 2002.

I convocated with my PhD in 2004 and was promoted to assistant professor also achieving tenure in the Faculty of Education at the University of Calgary. I received a lateral transfer to the Graduate Division of Educational Research to specialize in educational technology, where I was asked to develop a subspecialization in adaptive technologies. In addition to graduate student teaching and supervision, I teach our preservice teachers courses in inclusive education. I have a very rewarding career, which I believe comes from following your passions.

While I have presented my own autobiographical sketch here, this book would not exist if not for the conversations with many others, who brought their own histories and contexts to bear. In addition to the seven people who were primary informants for the *Blind Online Learners* inquiry highlighted in the pages to follow, my wonderful graduate student, Ania Paszuk and I conducted in-depth interactive interviews with 25 people to research this book. Most of the interviewees were blind. Other roles of the informants, sighted and blind, included parents, school board consultants, primary school teachers, postsecondary students, professors, researchers, and inventors and/or procurers of accessibility resources such as adaptive technologies. While all of the informants were remarkably generous with their time and their experiences, spending hours in conversation and being honest and forthright with their stories, particular gratitude must be extended to Dr. Bruce Clarke, Dr. Susan Crichton, Dr. Ron Ferguson, and to Marilyn Rushton. Doctors Clarke and Crichton supervised and advised the *Blind Online Learners* research. It was Dr. Ferguson who first invited me into this research domain, and his book, *We Know Who We Are*, that inspired me to try to write my own contribution to the field of blindness. Even though we are separated geographically, Marilyn and I developed a friendship that I treasure. She is a teacher, consultant, researcher, mother and friend—and she is blind. Both people served as metaphorical Jiminy Crickets on my shoulders. I hear their voices in my ears offering perspective on blindness throughout preparation of this text. Production of this book was supported through the generosity of the Professional Development and Research Institute on Blindness at Louisiana Tech University. In conjunction with their partner, the Louisiana Centre for the Blind, Institute on Blindness is *changing what it means to be blind.* The goal of this book is to contribute to this effort.

CHAPTER 1

BLINDNESS IS ABOUT VISION

The sighted majority's fascination with their visual experience makes the observations and insights of blind persons reflect outward even though visual impairment is a low incidence disability. In other words, while a very small minority will experience being blind, the rest of us will experience vision, and seeing, or not seeing, as the case may be, is a primary defining characteristic of who we are. Eye candy is a pillar of capitalism. Models, fashion, nail polish, hair color, glossy magazine advertising, billboards, and food dye would be unnecessary in a society constructed for the blind. Future spouses of most sighted persons have to pass the first, before they get that second glance, and the first minute of the job interview is in large part visual.

Vision upholds the primary aesthetic medium. In other words, most art forms are visual. Further, media such as photography, water color, and oil painting are not to be touched. Other arts such as performance art or theater can be multimedia, and are interactive, but are participatory for the performer and watched by the sighted viewer.

In our computer age, almost no attention has been paid to anything other than the visual interface. Try turning your monitor off and unplugging your mouse and using only your keyboard, even after downloading a trial version of screen reading software such as JAWS. Much of the Web is inaccessible and the information that is there is garbled and/or uninter-

Seeing Beyond Blindness, 1–15

esting. In most cases, it is laid out in a manner that makes it intriguing for the sighted, for example, in columns and tables, with photographs and images that screen readers (talking computers) cannot decipher. Sometimes, it is stripped down for a blind audience and then it is boring. Why should there not be interesting audio files, sound effects, and the like for those with hearing, just as there are interesting images, colors, headings, and white spaces for those with vision?

One needs to look no deeper than the external presentation of computers to realize that image is what counts. Not only do LCD (liquid crystal display) monitors maximize the visual display, they are aesthetic focal points. The black-rimmed LCD monitor is displayed on the work or home desk as if it were a bust of Beethoven on a grand piano. The bland yellowish hue of the hard-drive casing has been replaced by the aesthetically pleasing "desk-top." Beyond the monitors, the desk-tops and the peripherals like external drives and the sleek aerodynamic mouse are meant to be displayed. There is the power-suited all black design, the translucent blues and purples, and the IMAC proudly displaying its power-symbol high-tech guts.

In the rush of time that defines our modern pace, keeping your eyes on the goal is more than just a metaphor. Literal lack of vision results in illiteracy, unemployment, and poverty. Rates of Braille instruction are declining for qualified teachers and for children. Blind adults are less likely to enter and graduate from postsecondary institutions and to secure and maintain competitive employment, thus meaning poverty. Inaccessibility is interpreted as incompetence. It takes longer to study as a blind postsecondary student because you have to wait for electronic versions of the texts and produce Braille copies of the notes and papers for yourself and print for your instructors. You may be overlooked for employment because you have to rely on the inconvenience of public transportation.

Time is not just a barrier for the blind. Time is a power-laden cultural construct. Computer technology has redefined time. The result is a frenzy —an invented imperative to *fill* every moment, often resulting in metaphoric spinning tires. In the electronically connected Web of time we have little patience for waiting. The experience of aesthetics, computers, and time are not privy to those among us who are blind.

Postrel's (2003) treatise, *The substance of style*, on the place, role, and function of aesthetics in our lives reveals the same postulations as might a large-scale cultural ethnography of middle-class North Americans. By focussing on aesthetics, she captures the essence of being for many of us today. (No matter how uncomfortable or even distasteful this cultural portrait feels.) In other words, whether we like it or not, aesthetics is the central tent-pole and we have constructed such magnificent multiroomed awnings around it that try to disassemble the aesthetic pole and we would be smothered by the crashing structures and fabricated ceilings.

Aesthetics is more than beauty. Postrel (2003) explained, "it is the way we communicate through the senses" (p. 6). Aesthetics has a direct line to our consciousness without an intermediary. "It is the art of creating reactions without words, through the look and feel of people, places, and things." Postrel's thesis is that in this time and place in our lives, function and aesthetics are so tightly intertwined that there are no threads to separate. Historically, people have been interested in the dichotomy between form and function, substance and style. The discussion is dissolving as one is now so embedded in the other that to try to address them apart is nonsensical. However, this is not the way it has always been.

Rhetorical analysis conducted by communications historians reveals the scepticism with which "fancy" speeches were met. Public 'P'olitical addresses colored by figures of speech, metaphor, and pathos were dismissed as rhetoric, and the speakers as deceptive. It was perceived that there could not be logic and truth in aesthetically pleasing turns of phrase. Today, a politician would not dare to address an audience without a speech skilfully crafted by a speechwriter. For that matter, the primary broadcast medium being television, politicians are also not publicly presented without first being visually made-over. They require a new hairdo and dress-for-success lessons.

Academic research is no exception to the shift from separation of form and function to the collapsing of categories. The polar divides are melting. There was hard science and soft science. Objectivity of experimental research and disdain for what could not (shifted to *would* not) take that stance. Quantitative and qualitative research platforms, with the academics of the latter seeking acceptance by donning the epistemology of the former, were waved like divisive flags. Today, students design interdisciplinary degrees, creating links between fields such as physics and sociology, or biology and psychology. Medical scientists are engaging in interpretive research and seeking to apply the results. For example, an objective approach to teaching prospective doctors robotic bed-side manner gave way to ethnographies of hospitals and acknowledgement and respect for life perspective and humour.

Postman asserts that there are seldom new discoveries in human science. The importance of research about human relationships, experience, education, culture and the like is the telling of more revealing, engaging stories. The research is only as good as our ability to convey it and compel others to read it. In other words, the meaning of what we inquire into and present cannot be separated from the way in which it is languaged.

Postwar furniture was functional. With the contemporary taste for retro, bare-bones functional became fashion. In the reality television craze, many of the shows are dedicated to home improvement. Improving one's home means making it aesthetically pleasing. The functional tools are no exception to fashion. Postrel provided example after example of how everything from kitchen whisks to toilet bowl brushes, from sofas to refrigerators are now fashion accessories.

While Postrel's definition of aesthetics is sensory inclusive, the cultural examples are rarely. The senses include seeing, hearing, smelling, tasting, and touching. Yet it is the first that is dominant. The others are secondary. Consider Postrel's example of the overwhelming success of Starbucks coffee shops as an example. While there is something to be said for the smell and taste of the dark brew, that is not what compels people to spend disproportionately more than they would down the street at any other number of coffee shops. Do not underrate the aesthetic power of the coffee sleeve. I find myself asking for one if it is left off. It is not to protect my hand from the substance within, but to titillate and make me feel treated and even decadent. The interiors of Starbucks, even through the glance of the drive-through window, is skillfully planned to connote the whole cultural experience. From the "in" colors of the displayed refillable gadgeted to-go cups to the texture of the tiles, not felt through the feet but through the eye, everything is designed to please and to compel the return.

For those of us with sight, it goes beyond taking vision for granted. We love our vision and cannot fathom being without. We are visio-centric. Take for example, the cold empty thud of disappointment that comes with the response to the question—what do congenitally blind people dream? Somehow we expect that there must be some "escape" from the world of no visual images. At night-time when playful images dance in the mind's eye, surely the blind must be treated to the same pleasure? But of course, it is intuitive that at night, the blind experience the same sensory stimuli that they experience during their waking lives. During their REM (rapid eye movement) cycle, they experience voices, sounds, touches, feelings, emotions, sounds, and other such sensations, but not visual stimuli. Even more intuitive is that they do not grieve the absence of visual dreams any more than they grieve the absence of daytime sight, because not seeing is a blind person's reality.

Fear of losing our vision is deep-rooted and primordial. Ferguson (2001) presented a rigorous analysis of images of the blind through time. Whether to be interpreted as literal blinding, or figurative blocking of perception, punishment by taking away the power to see puts the fear of God into people. The references are biblical, and from the bible onwards, vision has been associated with light, and blindness with darkness. The dark is to be feared. There are unknown dangers lurking in the dark. The good guy rides away on the white stallion, and the bad guy wears the black Stetson and rides away on the black stallion to the sound of eerie music. Monsters and serial killers pop out of dark corners in horror movies. To be kept in the dark means to be denied knowledge and insight. *The Random House Dictionary* (1980) includes the following definitions of *dark*—"somber in hue," "gloomy or dismal," "evil or wicked," "ignorant or unenlightened," and "hidden or secret."

Titled "Egypt and Israel: Darkness and Light" Wisdom 17 in the Jerusalem Bible portrays terrible images of the punishment of darkness. The passage reads, "The whole world was shining with brilliant light and, unhindered, went on with its work; over them alone there spread a heavy darkness, image of the dark that would receive them." The passage goes on to describe their attempts to see, and when they cannot, the imaginings of monsters and their misinterpretation of the sounds around them. This darkness is portrayed as horrific. The men in the dark were "terrified." They were "prisoners of the dark," and "banished from eternal providence."

If you are sighted, close your eyes and what do you see? You see darkness. Try to walk around and attend to daily life and you are disoriented and crash into things. This is your experience of not having sight. This is not the blind person's experience. Eighty percent of people who are called blind are actually legally blind and have some vision. Even those who are totally blind do not see darkness. They see nothing. A quote from a blind person in a now forgotten source drives home this point. "I see through my eyes, what you see through your nose." With respect to bumping into things when we cannot use our eyes, this is also not the experience of blind people. Orientation and mobility training and practicing awareness of sounds, smells, and touch such as the proximity of objects means that blind people get around just fine. These facts are unknown and the linking of blindness and darkness is too strong and rests beneath our conscious awareness. Virginia Woolf wrote, "it is far more difficult to murder a phantom than a reality."

Until blindness is made salient for the sighted, the dominance of vision is not brought to conscious awareness. The sight bias is more insidious for its presence beneath our conscious awareness. Modernity was hailed and entrenched by the promise of science. Secular conversion to science yields the fruit of knowledge and with scientific research being the iron loop on which the keys to understanding all of the once-mysteries of our existence, science is perceived as the power to mastery of our universe. In order to experience that power we must have vision. Even though we cannot see the atom or the surface of the planets, vision gives us power to image it, to represent and thus manipulate (split/de-mortalize) it.

For some, postmodernism (elaborated in chapter 3) toppled the science idol. Scientific tenets are no longer privileged, and some renowned scientists described their works as explanatory stories—interpretations through treasured lenses. Vicious debate ensued. Anger and jealousy ensues when kicking in someone's well-crafted castle. In any case, the suspicions were raised. Science could no longer be the unquestioned omnipresent. Owens (1998) described the de-throning of visual privilege. Postmodern criticism,

> upsets the (modern) belief in vision as a privileged means of access to certainty and truth ("seeing is believing"). Modern aesthetics claimed that vision was superior to the other senses because of its detachment from its objects: "Vision," Hegel tells us in his *Lectures on Aesthetics*, "finds itself in a purely theoretical relationship with objects, through the intermediary of light, that immaterial matter which truly leaves objects their freedom, lighting and illuminating them without consuming them." ... For vision is hardly disinterested; nor is it indifferent, as Luce Irigaray has observed: "... In our culture, the predominance of the look over smell, taste, touch, hearing, has brought about an impoverishment of bodily relations ... The moment the look dominates, the body loses its materiality." That is, it is transformed into an image. (pp. 80-81)

Vision as the dominant and dominating sense has been unveiled by a small minority of academics and suspected in a confused hazy manner by others in the general populace. Vision as a key cultural construct remains largely undetected.

The leaves are starting to turn yellow, gold, and orange and the air is crisp. Summer is becoming a memory. One of the memories I hope a group of learners will hold of their summer is of a social constructionist approach to blindness. The course was specifically entitled *Developmental Aspects of Blindness*. It was one of those wonderful educational opportunities for me as a professor. There were many *aha!* moments. The students challenged one another, pushed one another's thinking and insightfully reflected. Yet, we discovered that sometimes the published literature is deficient, and no matter how hard many of the students tried, still a handful walked away parroting the dominant discourse.

Developmental psychology has been constructed by and for the mainstream populace and experimentation perpetuates the image of other as deficient. The sighted population is visio-centric and thereby the unconscious assumption holds that the only way that we can develop (i.e., learn) is through taking in visual stimuli. This includes seminal developmental psychologists such as Piaget. In other words, the developmental construct is visio-centric and the methodology is visually biased. Try to find developmental experimentation that authentically assesses development rather than vision. Consider, for example, the classic development experiments where two beakers of the same volume, one tall and skinny and the other short and squat are filled with water and children of various ages are asked to tell which holds more water. Consider, as another example, the experiment where a teddy bear is hidden behind a box to test awareness of object permanence. How are these concepts tested in the absence of vision? When one critically reads the literature, it becomes obvious that absence of vision becomes substituted for absence of development. If the construct cannot be tested, then it does not exist. The assumption is that if one cannot see, then one cannot develop/learn, so one is developmentally delayed/cognitively impaired. The red herring of it all is that this is confirmed in the research because the methodology is visually biased so that it looks like it is a scientific fact that blind children are developmentally delayed. With the power brand of the published sanction, authors such as Brambring and Troster (1994); Junefelt (2004); Levtzion-Korach, Tennenbaum, Schnitzer, and Ornay (2000); and Murdoch (1994) circulate the message to therapists, teachers, and through action conveyed to parents that blind children are fundamentally different and lesser—"performed worse" "significantly delayed" than sighted children. Celebrated authorities in the field of blindness, such as Dr. Kay Ferrell (1996) write that it is a matter of course that the development of visually impaired children differs from that of sighted children in both speed and type. Anecdotally, many of the adults interviewed for the background research of this text have secured graduate level degrees and demonstrate no indication of developmental delay. Many of the interviewed parents indicate no difference between the development of their sighted and blind sons and daughters provided that they, as parents, are creative in generating sensory experiential opportunities.

As researchers, it is incumbent upon us to remember to situate our data where it lives, not where it is convenient for us, or where tradition dictates.

> There was once an old man who was cold and shivering in the night. Beneath the light of a single street-light, he was hunched over on his hands and knees searching the pavement for a lost coin. Along came a younger man who offered to help look. The younger man said, "Show me just where you dropped it, and I will help you look." The older man pointed far across the street to where it was dark and said "I dropped it over there, but I wanted to search here where I had a chance of seeing it."

With respect to the example of developmental psychology, if we are expecting to find delays exhibited by blind children, then this is what our experimentation will probably reveal.

There is a natural fit between epistemology, ontology, and blindness. Many believe that the primary means of coming to know is through what we see with our own eyes. Further, that the test of what is real and true is what can be seen or measured by some means, even if our eyes require some external tool to enhance magnification. If we cannot observe first-hand because the sample size or population need be too large, or the field is too remote, then we can read the rigorous research of others and comfort ourselves with the reliability and validity of their methods. On the other hand, for those who believe that there is no external reality "out there" that exists apart from our contexts and perspectives, we want to read about the saturation of the research informants, the reflexivity of the researcher and the manner in which the interpretations were informed.

Magee (1995) was a philosopher who sought to explore ontology through the field of blindness. He thought if he could understand being blind, he could better understand who we are. He sought a correspondence with a fellow philosopher who was lacking what he considered to be the primary sense—vision. Magee's intention was to explore the limitations of his own senses through dialogue with a blind philosopher. Magee believes that all humans are deprived of sensory knowledge through the limitations of our phenomenology. Some people have the senses of sight, hearing, touch, taste, and smell. We receive the world around us through these senses. Magee believes that there is much to the world beyond the reality that we can comprehend. We simply do not have the senses to receive or even imagine the other facets. He wanted to explore these limitations through conversation with a philosopher who did not have the *primary* receptive capacity-vision.

In 1995 a series of letters between Magee and Milligan was published as a text. The text is powerful. It is a correspondence between two scholars, both of whom lived a political reality, and pondered metaphysics within their departments of philosophy. As such it is illuminating. It was written in the voice of the sighted and the voice of the blind.

Magee started out uninformed about blindness. He did not comprehend the tension between the organized blind and professional agencies when he sought out a correspondence with a blind philosopher (Milligan) regarding metaphysics and the limitations of human senses. To Magee's initial frustration, the two philosophers needed to dialogue regarding beliefs about blindness, social positioning, and political ramifications prior to engaging in metaphysical discussion. Magee began the correspondence with an unstated assumption that he believed was a moot point. He believed that life must be experienced as radically and profoundly different for blind-from-birth individuals. He believed that blind people were sensory-deprived and that their lack of vision was tragic. As informant, Milligan served to inform both Magee and the readers privy to their correspondence.

Milligan, the blind philosopher, was aligned with the National Federation of the Blind. Americans belonging to the National Federation of the

Blind, an organized group of blind citizens, do not see themselves as having a disability. That is not to say that they do not see themselves as disadvantaged, stigmatized, or oppressed. They believe that the source of the disability rests within society, not with the blind individual. Further, blindness is not a tragedy. Blind persons are not to be rescued, pitied, or admired.

Milligan's response incorporated both political and metaphysical perspective. He stated that blind people are normal human beings who happen not to be able to see. The sighted are challenged to "look beyond" a love for vision, to "see" that the world can be comprehended through the other senses. Milligan argued that we communicate, name, and mediate reality through language. Further, all language is propositional. We construct phenomena through the words we use to communicate about them. As such, the world is experientially the same for the blind as it is for the sighted. Such communication, however, depends upon opportunity of experience. For example, the sighted and the blind can communicate about a tree both pragmatically and metaphorically provided that both have experienced trees through seeing them or touching them, and talking and hearing about them. Unfortunately, the conversation was truncated when Milligan died, giving Magee the last, but self-recognized as incomplete—final word.

If, as Milligan believed, we mediate the world through words, are the experiences of blind people essentially the same as the sighted? Helen Keller's experience makes an interesting case in this regard. Notably, Helen Keller was blind and deaf. Through a manual finger language, Annie Sullivan, Helen Keller's teacher, read a great deal of literature to Helen as a primary teaching strategy (Herrmann, 1998). Herrmann presented Helen as ravenous for language upon being introduced to symbolic communication. She loved literature, memorized it, and adopted it as her own. Helen's own writings are filled with poetic visual depictions, such as those describing the colors of the rainbow and the clouds on the mountaintops. Being blind, Helen cannot have had first-hand sensory experience of these phenomena. As a young girl, Helen endured a plagiarism hearing for replicating a story and presenting it as her own. Helen claimed no recollection of ever having heard the story. Herrmann supported the theory that the so-called plagiarism was actually an incident arising from verbalism (experiences mediated through words rather than direct sensory experience). The public incident sparked debates regarding whether Helen's writing and even her experience of the world were mimicry or original.

In his book titled *Writing in the Dark*, van Manen (2002) explored the relationship between direct sensory experience, language, consciousness, and research. He shared an interpretation of the story of Orpheus and

Eurydice from classical mythology. Hamilton (1942) retold this tale. Orpheus made beautiful music on his lyre and no woman could resist him. He chose Eurydice to be his bride, but right after the wedding ceremony while still in her gown, she was bitten by a viper and died. Orpheus was so desperate to have Eurydice back that he went down to the "underworld" to retrieve her. He charmed the guards with his music and the gods "who rule the dark [another testament to the discussion of dark and light above] and silent world" made a deal with him (p. 109). He could have his bride back, but on one condition. She was to follow him up the path to the living, but he could not look back at her until they were both "in the light." Here is what happened.

> He knew that she must be just behind him, but he longed unutterably to give one glance to make sure. But now they were almost there, the blackness was turning gray; now he had stepped out joyfully into the daylight. Then he turned to her. It was too soon; she was still in the cavern. He saw her in the dim light, and he held out his arms to clasp her; but on the instant she was gone. She had slipped back into the darkness. All he heard was one faint word, "Farewell." (p. 109)

With respect to the meaning of this mythology, on a superficial level, one can reflect on delayed gratification and Orpheus' inability to wait, or his deep love for Eurydice causing him to forget his promise. However, the allusions to light and dark, with their primordial associations, push our interpretations deeper. van Manen explored a literary meaning.

Consider Orpheus as writer, as researcher, as artist. Eurydice is who he wants to know. She is the object of his gaze. In the stark light of day, what she appears to be gets in the way of knowing who she truly is. Aesthetics are like a Mobious loop because they focus on the external appearance and yet evoke our unconscious. Postrel (2003) wrote,

> Whatever information aesthetics conveys is prearticulate—the connotation of the color and shapes of letters, not the meanings of the words they form. Aesthetics conjures meaning in a subliminal, associational way, as our direct sensory experience reminds us of something that is absent, a memory or an idea. (p. 6)

The interpretive researcher seeks to observe and understand, and yet is confined to the language of words to describe what is experienced. To write a poem "as lovely as a tree" is the goal, and yet it is impossible. The language of words is not complex enough. The interpretive researcher longs to be postliterate. In turning to look at Eurydice while she is still in the tunnel of darkness, Orpheus was seeking to see her "before she resumed her mortal state" (van Manen, 2002, p. 242). He longed to see "the true being of love, to see Eurydice in her pure invisibility." van Manen explained,

> The artist tries to bring things into presence through artistic evocation. But to see the being of things directly would require that, like Orpheus, one moves into that space where the invisibility of the real has not yet compromised itself into visible form. It is here, in this realm of "wild being" that things exist, before they have gotten names attached to them, before they can hide themselves behind words. It happens that in this wondering gaze one may suddenly "recognize" the fragility of human understanding, to see existence in its naked appearance, to peer past the veneer of human constructs. (p. 243)

The interpretive researcher seeks phenomenological experience—to record life steeped in meaning as humans are engaging in their everyday journey of being. Yet, human experience is mediated through language. For example, when interviewing someone, there are the layers of language as intermediary. First, there are the words that someone has been told about oneself—some chosen, some unconsciously accepted, others chewed on and spit out. Does *extravert* with all of its connotations describe the being of the wearer? Then there are the words the interviewee chooses to tell the story. The line weaves between the public and private self. The interviewee's story is veiled through the chosen words. The story is not being experienced on-the-spot. How are our experiences storied and whose truth are they? What of the interviewee's vocabulary? Do the words tell the story that is in the heart? Then there is the space between what the interviewee is telling and what the interviewer is hearing. Each has lived a different life until now, thus giving the words different associations.

Returning now to the discussion of Helen Keller as writer, what does being blind (and in her case also deaf) mean with regard to the nature of her experience? Using the mythology of Orpheus and Eurydice, ironically Keller might be interpreted as being trapped in the *light*. She was confined to the world of words with no possibility of being able to enter the underworld to *write in the dark*. Without being able to see or hear directly, she could only mediate experience through the veil of what others wrote or said about the phenomena. In her phenomenology of drawing, Montgomery-Whicher (2002) inquired into the aesthetic experience. She wrote,

> *Seeing* has connotations of knowledge as well as sight. For example, we say "I see" when we understand something, and the word "insight" suggests a mode of knowing in which one sees into the nature of things. As I pick up my pen and resume drawing, my seeing slides into "seeing" in spite of my effort to maintain a cool dispassionate gaze, calculating angles, mentally measuring this width against that length. As my eyes scrutinize my sister's face, I suddenly "see" her: I see her face with my eyes and my seeing sees

> through the face she shows to the world. My relationship with my sister is intensified by being temporarily suspended.... In this silent conversation conducted between my eye, my hand and her face, between my pen and paper, I see her, I meet her. (p. 41)

This passage is philosophical and yet built upon the constructions of the commonplace. As a sighted majority, we assume that those who have no vision cannot *see*.

What of the sighted? Are we in-sight? Do we have insight? As a culture, we are trapped in Orpheus' light. Television and movies have propagated aesthetic images serving as icons to be adopted and consumed by the public. The marketed images are entrenched by their capitalistic capacity. Industries such as cosmetics and cosmetic surgery, clothing retail, and furniture manufacture are built upon visual predilection. The financial arrangements make certain that advertising budgets keep the images in circulation.

The celebration of the image has had consequences. Naomi Wolf's (2002) edition of her book *The Beauty Myth: How Images Of Beauty Are Used Against Women*, explains that 11 years after her original edition, the beauty myth had expanded so that there is also a male beauty myth. The beauty myth is that there is an ideal image to aspire to at any cost. Flip through any magazine or channel hop, and we see only air brushed *perfection*—for women this means young, extremely thin, and preferably White-skinned and blonde. Wolf explained that the beauty myth has taken its insidious place in a series of "cultural conspiracies."

> Other such fictions arose contemporaneously: a version of childhood that required continual maternal supervision; a concept of female biology that required middle-class women to act out the roles of hysterics and hypochondriacs; a conviction that respectable women were sexually anesthetic; and a definition of women's work that occupied them with repetitive, time-consuming, and painstaking tasks such as needlepoint and lacemaking. (p. 15)

Wolf explained that just as these preceding myths were collusions to control women's behavior, so too is the beauty myth. She provided elaborated example after example of the beauty myth's impacts such as heightening competition between women and keeping women powerless as we suffer the insecurities of our imperfect shells.

Celebration of aesthetics as a cultural conspiracy yields a counter-interpretation regarding the *deficiencies* of the blind. A note of caution here, in that blind citizens are not above the insidious unconscious socially constructed collusions of our culture. Blind people are victim to the same myths such as that beauty is to be elevated above other values (and that it is a value at all). That being said, is it possible that being blind enables escape from the domination of the visual superficial? Does not being able to see allow the salience of what matters? Boman (2002) titled her book *Ex-Sighted, A New Vision* to capture this experiential unshackling. Her interviews with numerous individuals who were previously sighted and became legally blind derived a common theme, in that the interviewees shared a new life perspective on what matters and what does not. They no longer bought into the importance of physical beauty in the way in which we value ourselves and others. They no longer craved material possessions simply for their prettiness and thereby status.

When I am at a conference watching a series of speakers, I long to shut off my stream of consciousness inner voice with its commentary on the hairstyles, clothing choice, figure, and posture of the women presenters. I long to hear only their presentation without the veil of their visual image. This is the honest reflection of a highly educated fellow woman. Returning to the mythology of Orpheus and Eurydice, perhaps Helen Keller was not trapped in the light of words, but had a passageway to the transcendent meaning where Eurydice remained. Perhaps Helen was not distracted by the look or even the sound of people's voices and could therefore more directly experience the essence of phenomena. Surely as defined as an unconscious awakening, aesthetics are not the exclusive domain of the sighted.

Pondering the relationship between Keller's external or sensory experience and her internal or interpretive, psychological, constructive, and aesthetic experience leaves us with many questions. Due to her blindness and deafness and her teacher's methods, Helen's primary experience of language and its association with the world around her was through the authored word. Are mental pictures equivalent to visual pictures and if so, is the use of metaphor effective in educational contexts? Are metaphors predominantly visual or can they be equivalently interpreted through other senses?

How paramount is experience to reception of visual images? Deborah (one of the research informants, whose story is shared in chapter 5) described her mother's influence on Deborah's perception of the world around her. Deborah's mother constantly and consistently described images to her. When Deborah's mother dressed her, she explained that Deborah was wearing a white dress with a blue sash with matching white patent shoes with blue bows. When evening approached, Deborah's mother took her outside and described the colors of the sunset. If images are often and fully described to a blind child, are his experiences of educational images different than for someone who did not receive this description? If so, in what way? It has been suggested that blind people may better attain and retain focus, because with the absence of visual stimuli, they are less prone to what Mayer (2001) presented as the capacity-limitation hypothesis (p. 152), or in other words, sensory and even cognitive overload. Can this be empirically substantiated? Where do images described in words "fit" in terms of multimedia cognitive theory? Are they words or are they pictures? Are binary communication channels an accurate depiction? Finally, is there a difference in terms of cognitive processing between reading text on the computer monitor and hearing it through screen reading software?

Since Wileman's (1980) publication of his book, *Exercises in Visual Thinking*, the mechanism to produce and display visual educational aides has changed, while the underlying stance has not. Wileman's text explicates and illustrates strategies in visually depicting facts, processes, theories and numerical data. His publication date preceded the widespread personal computer era that empowered most educators to be desktop publishers, including searching catalogues of clipart as illustrations. His directions to use pen and ink and transparencies has long been surpassed by the advent of Microsoft Powerpoint and LCD projectors.

The imperative for visual representation has not changed. The user-friendly techniques to make and display the image presentation (even by the blind for the sighted) has further entrenched the visual expectation. Neither Wileman (1980) nor reader questioned the untested assumption that people learn better when words, numbers and concepts are accompanied by visual images. The book title is *Visual Thinking* even though the book does not delve beyond mechanistic instructional technology to explore the cognitive processes that occur when internally visualizing and interpreting the world around us. One does not need vision to engage in internal organization of phenomena. However, it is taken as a given that only the sighted internally represent.

Ask someone who has not recently been pondering sight and blindness to define "reading." In my own casual experiments, seeing is almost always fundamental to the definition. Consider Wileman's (1980) definition of reading—"seeing with the eyes and understanding that which is seen" (p. 12). It is only our "retinal chauvinism" that causes us to believe that we need to see to read. People who are feeling Braille dots are reading. I define reading as—deciphering symbols to attain meaning. Blind readers, including those who are blind from birth, have access to recorded words and numbers and the meanings that these symbols convey. They have means of internally representing the form and figure of the symbols as well as the conveyed concrete and abstract meanings. Our language allows us to internally represent memories, feelings and imaginings that are not immediately available to our senses. This ability is the domain of the sighted and the blind. It is only our visual predilection that assumes that one needs to see in order to read, learn, and even think.

My mother sat on a chair behind me while I interviewed my friend Marilyn. Marilyn is a "vision teacher," consulting to blind and visually impaired children as well as their teachers and parents throughout a school division. Marilyn is a role model for the children as she herself is blind. My Mom asked to sit in on the interview, as she is a retired school teacher and spent the latter years prior to retirement as a resource teacher consulting regarding "special needs." The two women discovered another connection prior to the interview while I set up my equipment and Marilyn showed Mom around her home. They stopped at the piano. Marilyn is a musician and Mom did a music sabbatical. Prior to the interview, I coached Mom that she would have to remain silent so that I could use the audiovideo clips for a course I was developing. However, when Marilyn said that she is a *visual learner,* Mom audibly caught her breath and then said, "You can't possibly mean that. Do you mean that you think in words? Or images?" To provide some further context, my Mom, who is sighted, is very definitely an auditory learner. She has quite a remarkable ability to hear a piece of music once and proceed to play it on the piano with little difficulty without the sheet music. Marilyn explained that she considers Braille to be very important to her because she cannot study without it. Marilyn has a masters level degree and despite the cumbersome nature of Braille due to the voluminous size, Marilyn embosses all of her papers, texts, and notes so that she can see them. In her mind's eye, she sees Braille dots. She is a visual learner. This contrasts with my sighted Mom, for whom music has always come easier than writing narrative.

My own learning style contrasts with that of Marilyn. I had a good chunk of this chapter written in my mind's eye before the black loops, circles, and lines started appearing on my monitor. I stared at the empty white space framed by the fancy LCD monitor and wondered about the threat of translating those thoughts that sounded profound in-here-onto-there and was it the worry of making them look good or sound good that worried me. Do blind people transcend this pettiness? I had an hour long in-my-head conversation with Max van Manen (2002) about his serendipitously named book *Writing In The Dark* agreeing that "Yes, Max, writing is difficult," before I could overcome my temporary paralysis and begin. All this, and on a morning self-described to my husband as a "writerly" mood. I hope that these words put you in a writerly mood and require you to extend what has not been said, and that you have a conversation with the me that is present in the words that I have put down on these pages.

CHAPTER 2

IMAGES OF BLINDNESS

INTRODUCTION

The Canadian National Institute for the Blind's (CNIB) *Living With Vision Loss: A Handbook for Caregivers* opens with a quotation, "more people are blinded by definition than by any other cause" (p. 1). In other words, the stigma of blindness (while taken for granted and applied unconsciously in day-to-day cultural interchanges) is not inevitable. Disability studies scholars argue that the *idea* of blindness and the matrix of interactions have come into being culturally and historically, or in other words, are socially constructed (Asch, 1995; Ferguson, 2001; Marks, 1999; Scott, 1969; Shapiro, 1993). Blindness research is shaped by and even built upon assumptions and prejudices. As such, efforts to contribute to new knowledge in the field of blindness can only be understood and navigated through an examination of the historical applications of blindness research and the implications on power and status.

This chapter defines and critiques "social construction" within the context of blindness. The ontological and epistemological properties of blindness are argued, and the definition of legal blindness considered. The positioning of blind people within Canadian and U.S. contemporary culture is shared as documented by constructionists, and the challenging voice as lodged through the (U.S.) National Federation of the Blind

Seeing Beyond Blindness, 17–37

(NFB) recognized. The current year of papers from the primary journal—*Journal of Visual Impairment and Blindness* (JVIB)—presenting and informing the theory of academics and the practice of professionals is analyzed. Because the research explicated in this text concerns online learning, the NFB's position on educational technology is quoted, with an interpretation of some of the historical precedents and principles as antecedents to that position.

Critique of Social Constructionism

Hacking (1999) defines constructionism as "various sociological, historical, and philosophical projects that aim at displaying or analyzing actual, historically situated, social interactions or causal routes that led to, or were involved in, the coming into being or establishing of some present entity or fact" (p. 8). Applied to the field of blindness, this definition means that researchers use actual documents such as records of correspondence, text books, works of art and meeting minutes to analyze the meaning given to blindness (in a specified time and place) and the implications on the social positioning of blind people. Hacking is direct and transparent about his disdain for the label-social construction. He wrote,

> I have seldom found it helpful to use the phrase "social construction" in my own work. When I have mentioned it I have done so in order to distance myself from it. It seemed to be both obscure and overused. Social construction has in many contexts been a truly liberating idea, but that which on first hearing has liberated some has made all too many others smug, comfortable, and trendy in ways that have become merely orthodox. The phrase has become code. If you use it favorably, you deem yourself rather radical. If you trash the phrase, you declare that you are rational, reasonable, and respectable. (p. vii)

Hacking *does* believe (and illustrates in his own writings) that many of the unconscious beliefs humans hold about phenomena are not inevitable, that they are shaped through the context of time and place, and that some of these should and can be altered through use of explicit language and oftentimes action. However, Hacking finds the metaphor unsuitable, the linking of the two words redundant, the phenomenon of the inquiry overgeneralized, and the term politicized as it has come to represent academic turf-wars.

The unfortunate metaphor and its linking of "social" and "construction" as well as the failure to designate the phenomenon of inquiry in much social constructionist writing necessitates further discussion. Construction is the practice of building up from raw materials; it connotes images of manual labor and tools. This is problematic in that some theorists argue that there are no "social" raw materials (Magee & Millian, 1995, p. 116), in that all discursive acts are subject to interactivity and intertextuality; phenomena are defined in a context rather than discretely (Alvesson & Sköldberg, 2000; Franklin, 1999; Haraway, 1998; Usher, 1996). Second, images of laborers showing up in designated spots, at prearranged times, wearing tool-belts implies intentionality. The "building" as noun is the intent of the "building" as verb. Yet, while the unearthing and analysis of social constructionists is deliberate and intentional, the discursive acts and implications of social institutions are often not. Marks (1999) provided the example that human service agencies and their professionals do not deliberately set out to oppress. Finally, Hacking (1999) wrote, adding "social" to the metaphor of "construction" is usually redundant. One of his examples was that, of course, policy and conversation are social; they could not exist if not for the interactions of people.

The crux of Hacking's (1999) question (privileged as the title of his text)—*The Social Construction of What?* is a differentiation and explicit identification of phenomena given by the laws of nature versus phenomena shaped culturally and historically through the language and practices of humans. Not being able to see is not socially constructed. The *idea* of blindness, on the other hand, and the whole matrix of human service organizations including educational institutions; attitudes and cultural practices toward blind citizens; and policies—are socially constructed. In the words of tenBroek (1957), "the origin of the disability is plainly inside the blind person [nature-given]. The origin and responsibility for the handicap are just as plainly outside him—in the attitudes and preconceptions of the community" (p. 6). Failing to distinguish, spawns a red herring for opponents to social construction, thus hurting the cause of consciousness raising.

Marks (1999) lodged three criticisms of social construction—when applied to disability. Her criticisms are in the context of social constructionism as consciousness raising, or in other words, efforts of the organized disabled to unmask oppression. First, social constructionists are charged with a limiting perspective that fails to account for diversity. Accounts of what constitutes physical barriers, for example, are said to be defined by "white, Western, male wheelchair users" (p. 87). Marks noted discontent from those with cognitive or sensory impairments, such as blindness, for the underrepresentation of their diverse experiences.

Second, and intertwined with the first criticism, the disabled social movement fails to "trouble" ideals of capitalism, particularly exemplified by the support of the rehabilitative return-to-work goals. An example might be drawn from the presentation of Scott's (1969) text in which the characteristics attributed to blind people were "helplessness, dependency, melancholy, docility, gravity of inner thought, [and] aestheticism" (p. 4). None of these ways of being are inherently negative, and yet in Western culture, independence and self-reliance are escalated above dependence and helplessness, and extraversion is valued over melancholy, docility, and gravity of inner thought, and pragmatism considered more desirable than aestheticism (Dossa, 1990).

As described below, the primary distinction between Scott's (1969) and Ferguson's (2001) texts lies in the focus on the blindness agencies of the first, and the organized blind of the second. Even while questioning the day-to-day practice and outcomes of blindness agencies, Scott did not question the notion of the human service institution, and in fact recommended strategies for its amelioration. Ferguson, on the other hand, does not take as "given" that blindness presents a social problem, and thereby does not assume that blindness agencies are a natural resolution.

Finally, "disability," as the unifying theme or matrix, is problematic in its definition. Activists reject the imposed definitions that are constructed largely through the medical profession. This leaves a troubling empty space in the collective quest necessary to unify the participants. It is replaced by "identity." In other words, self-identification as disabled is the definitional qualification. Marks explained that this oversimplifies notions of identity. Goffman's (1959) text describes the complexity of self-understanding and self-presentation, such that rather than having and displaying a "core unified self" (i.e., suggested here to include the stable role as "disabled"), persons are highly variable and self-identify according to the context. As described below in the context of positions on technology, the question of identity as blind can be conflictual for those with low or no vision. Blindness agencies have a history of informing the blind that they need to take on a new identity if they lose their vision, once having had it (Asch, 1995; Ferguson, 2001; Scott, 1969). Blind advocates disagree. The affiliation with organized groups such as the National Federation of the Blind has been found to improve the social situation of blind citizens, and yet as described by Asch (1995), Ferguson, and Jernigan (1963/1990, 1965), blind people, as a rule, do not equivocate themselves to a culture, but consider themselves to be "normal" citizens.

Blindness—Defined/Constructed

Blindness is a condition of ontological objectivity and epistemological subjectivity (to borrow and apply the terminology of Searle (1995), to a new context). Ontology is the study of the nature of existence. Epistemology is the study of how we come to know. Searle's use of the word *objective* means that something exists through the laws of nature. It does not rely on language for its existence. As the converse, the word *subjective* means that something exists as a construct; humans have named and attempted to create a shared meaning for a phenomenon. As examples, a mountain is "objective;" a mountain is a looming mass of rock that exists whether humans name it "mountain" or "bizzwhit." The naming does not change the nature of its being. The game of hockey is "subjective." If not for the rules that humans have agreed upon, the game would not exist. That there are three periods, what counts as offside, and how many players are allowed on the ice at one time, are not laws of nature. There is no such thing as hockey beyond human invention, despite the fact that the fan appeal is just as real as the blood oozing from the player's face following a fight.

For something to be ontologically objective means that its existence is present through the laws of nature. Whatever we call it—however we talk about it - whatever metaphorical significance we assign to it—its existence is indisputable and determinate. If, on the other hand, something is ontologically subjective, it exists only through the creation of people. This is not to say that the experience of it is fictive or imaginary like a unicorn or leprechaun—even though some dispute the existence of some constructions such as Fibromyalgia. Ontological subjectivity means that something exists because people have put language to it and thereby given it meaning. One can change the laws constructed by people (despite long and arduous processes). One cannot change the laws of nature.

The game of hockey was described above as subjective. This is to say that it is ontologically subjective—it would not exist if humans had not had the idea for the game and then drew up the rules for its play. At the same time, the game of hockey is epistemologically objective. Players wearing skates and pads, wielding sticks used to provide momentum to a puck is indisputably the game of hockey. It does not matter that the rules differ between the Olympic and the national league manifestation, or that different languages have different terms for the game—humans have constructed a shared understanding that this sport with these certain signifiers is the game of hockey. Epistemological subjectivity, on the other hand, means that how we come to know about something is through the languaged meaning subscribed to it by people.

The phenomenon of blindness is ontologically objective. The experience of being blind is very real; a blind person must be very close up to see, has minimal peripheral vision, or cannot see at all. There is no phenomenological doubt in the condition. tenBroek's (1957) address reads,

> let me be very clear about this. I have no wish to minimize the character and extent of blindness as a disability. It is for all of us a constant nuisance and a

> serious inconvenience. To overcome it requires effort and patience and initiative and guts. (p. 6)

On the other hand, the way in which we "know" that someone is blind, or in other words, their designation as "legally blind" exists only in the "rules and practices of people" (Hacking, 1999, p. 30). Blindness is epistemologically subjective. Scott (1969) presented and critiqued the definition of blindness. He explained that the definition exists "for the purpose of determining eligibility for services to the blind" (p. 40). Scott cited the American Foundation for the Blind's (1967) definition of blindness. He quoted the definition as,

> Central visual acuity of 20/200 or less in the better eye, with correcting lenses; or central visual acuity of more than 20/200 if there is a field defect in which the peripheral field has contracted to such an extent that the widest diameter of visual field represents an angular distance no greater than 20 degrees. (p. 40)

To interpret this definition, a person with 20/20 vision can read the entire ophthalmologist's (Snellen) eye-chart from 20 feet away. The person with 20/200 vision can see at 20 feet away from the Snellen chart, what the person with 20/20 vision can see at 200 feet away. In terms of angular distance, side-vision might be impaired at the inner and/or outer "corner" of the eye. Whereas a person who is legally blind has less than 20 degrees of outer angular distance, a person with normal vision has over 200 degrees of peripheral vision.

The assigning of the number 20/200 as a decision line is a construction of people. It can be altered. If for example, the incidence of blindness overcame the financial resources allocated to supporting people with this condition, the number could be changed to 20/400. In other words, a person is only classified as legally blind if he can see at 20 feet away, what a person with 20/20 vision can see at 400 or more meet away. Suddenly, all of the people who have 20/200 vision would find themselves ineligible for supports even though their challenges had not decreased. This very practice occurred in the field of cognitive impairment when the decision lines designated by intelligence quotients were shifted.

Texts Within the Context of Blindness

As well as the very definition of what counts as blindness being subjective, so too are the positioning of blind people in our culture and the services structured to provide supports that blind people are constructed to require. Three texts are reviewed to examine the "image" of blindness.

The first, *The Making of Blind Men* by Robert A. Scott (1969) is one of the foundational texts in both blindness and disability studies, as it is an empirical study of the "disability of blindness [as] a learned social role" (p. 14). While Scott's text is framed in the context of human services for the blind, or what Scott called "blindness agencies," the second text presented here, *We Know Who We Are* by Ronald J. Ferguson (2001) embraces the perspective of the organized blind. His is a reflexive interpretation of the history of social policy and educational practice. Moshe Barasch's (2001) *Blindness: The History of a Mental Image in Western Thought* differs from the preceding two primarily in its source materials; Barasch analyzed literary works and visual arts such as paintings and sculptures produced in Antiquity, Early Christianity, the Middle Ages, the Renaissance and the Enlightenment. He used these images to explore how the blind were imagined.

The Making of Blind Men by Robert A. Scott (1969)

While Hacking (1999) might happily note that Scott (1969) does not use the term "social construction" in his title or throughout his text, Scott's thesis follows the two main propositions outlined by Hacking as constituting the construct. In keeping with the first proposition, Scott's thesis is that the stigmatizing characteristics as exhibited by and/or wrongfully attributed to blind people through stereotypy, are not "given by nature," or in other words, are not primary characteristics of blindness. What are the personality and emotional characteristics associated with blindness? Scott identified these attributes as "helplessness, dependency, melancholy, docility, gravity of inner thought, [and] aestheticism" (p. 4). In keeping with the second proposition of social construction, Scott considered these associations as taken-for-granted, or in other words, considered to be commonsense by the general public.

Scott (1969) collected empirical evidence through interviews, observations, and analysis of historical documents to demonstrate how "the blind character" has been acquired (in the perception of the public, and even in the actions of many blind people) through cultural practices, largely in the form of the human-service institution. The evidence that Scott interpreted in support of his propositions can be summarized in three points. First, Scott identified a pattern whereby blind people are "rewarded" for assimilating the beliefs of the experts and playing the role of "good" clients, and "punished" for acting otherwise. Second, the rehabilitative practices of most agencies reinforce conditions leading to a life of dependence and compliance. Most agencies *voice* a philosophy of "restoration" characterized by a belief that "blind people can lead independent and fulfilled lives in the outside world" (p. 119). At the same time, most *practice* a limiting type of accommodative rehabilitation that regards the restorative goals as "noble" but "unrealistic" (p. 119). Third, the social presentation of blind people who are not in service of blindness agencies is markedly different. Scott wrote, "these people, particularly blinded veterans and the independent blind, fail to display the attitudinal and behavioral patterns that so many insist they should have because they are blind" (p. 120).

Hacking (1969) identified six gradations of constructionism (p. 19). The grades are listed in order of increasing distaste for the status quo and in increasing social action, to where action might be described as aggressive. The gradations are: historical, ironic, reformist or alternatively unmasking, rebellious, and revolutionary. Hacking distinguished between the metaphors of "unmasking" and "revealing" or "exposing," explaining that what the word "unmasking" adds to the latter two is "an overtone of exposing something that was deliberately covered, in order to conceal its true nature" (p. 53).

Scott's (1969) text operates at the level of unmasking, demonstrating the author's belief that consciousness-raising holds the potential to effect great change, particularly within a human institution that seems to yield influence, such as the blindness agency. Scott was unmasking rather than revolutionizing; he did not want to take a metaphorical wrecking-ball to blindness agencies. In fact, he believed that conscious and critical application of their influential resources can yield positive advances in the social positioning and status of the blind. He wrote,

> Some may regard as deplorable the fact that blindness agencies have so great an impact upon the very nature of the phenomenon of blindness in our society. I do not, for it suggests this system has the potential of becoming a powerful tool for positive social change.... Blind men are not born, they are made; the challenge to an organized intervention system such as work for the blind is to render the process by which this occurs both rational and deliberate. The first step that must be taken in order to transform the current system from a tool with uncertain and unintended consequences for the blind it purportedly serves into one that can be used for positive social change is to reexamine and critically evaluate the scientific validity of blindness workers' assumptions about blindness and the blind. (p. 121)

Scott's formula for reformation is unlikely to be successful for three reasons. First, Scott asserted that blind people in the service of agencies tend to act in conformity with the expectations of the agencies. Thus, "reexamination" through observing people who are acting in confirmatory ways will only reinforce previously held beliefs. Second, as described by Goffman (1963) stigma (impaired relationships with those who are undesirable/discredited) is a powerful phenomenon in that the stigmatized are seen as "not quite human" (p. 5). Stigma is not easily shed, at least in part because of a further phenomenon that Hacking (1969) called "interactivity"; blind people see themselves as they are seen by others (Jernigan, 1963/1990, 1965). Third, the "rational" and "deliberate" rendering of constructive processes is naïve and unrealistic, and unless strong tools of analysis and contrary constructions show that the stigma of blindness and the interactive effects on blind people are not "given by nature" or inherent to blindness and to our social ways of being, no progress in effecting change in the societal status of blind people can be hoped for.

While Scott's (1969) text has been used here to exemplify the empirical application of social constructionism within the context of blindness, (and it is beyond the scope of this chapter to present an extensive critique of this single text), it would be incongruent with the text's theme of consciousness-raising to leave some of the problems from a critical theoretical perspective unidentified. First, the title and all gendered pronouns throughout the text are masculine. The term "men" is insensitive to gender and thereby power relations. Second, just as the organized blind were not invited to inform the beliefs and practices of the blindness agencies, so too was this source of empirical inspiration ignored by Scott. He did not give even passing mention to the organized blind such as the early National Federation of the Blind. This oversight is unfortunate, as it would have facilitated the incorporation of multiple voices, and challenging ones at that. It is reasonable to expect that the philosophy and perspective of the organized blind would have resulted in a profile in stark contrast to the one of helplessness, docility, and dependence, and thus would have fuelled Scott's thesis that these behaviors were "pulled" from the institutional system.

We Know Who We Are by Ronald J. Ferguson (2001)

This text is unique within the body of literature in two main ways—first, in its conceptualization and mechanism of policy studies, and second, in its alignment with the organized blind. Traditional policy studies view both "social ills" and approaches to their amelioration as historical truths to be traced and analyzed (Scheurich, 1994). Postmodern approaches "strip" the solutions of their "authority" and trouble their truth value, but fail to trouble the particular problems and/or the very construction of social phenomena as a 'problem' or metaphorical "ill." Ferguson's (2001) policy archaeology, on the other hand, questions the "givenness" of the social problem, the means by which the phenomena becomes socially visible, the construction of the various solutions, and even the social functions of policy studies.

The second, and interrelated departure is in authoring perspective. Within traditional blindness literature, the archives sought and the social and educational history presented (thereby given written primacy and status) has been overwhelmingly that of the national professional agencies and organizations. Ferguson (2001), on the other hand, rigorously traced the development of the National Federation of the Blind, analyzing the social and educational policies and practices necessitating its inception, the counter-forces barring its formation until 1940, and the fortitude of the people who finally brought it to its contemporary position of influence with a membership of over 50,000.

The primary sources inspiring Ferguson's (2001) method of policy archaeology were Michel Foucault's (1972) *The Archaeology of Knowledge* and James Scheurich's (1994) "Policy archaeology: A new policy studies methodology." Ferguson began his text with a chapter describing policy archaeology and applying it to the history of education of the blind. To take a very small extract from Ferguson's carefully constructed chapter on his methodology, "archaeology is an attempt to understand how discourses are developed and how discourses place constraints on thought and behavior" (p. 6). Ferguson quoted Foucault's definition of discourse as "organized bodies of knowledge and practice, such as clinical medicine" (p. 5). Strathern (2000) explained that for Foucault (1972-1977), discourse is a culture-specific application in the form of "concepts, practices, and statements" originating in the epistemes, or mind-set of the age. Policy archaeology might be understood as a systematic study of what "counts" as a social problem, and the social construction of solutions through recovery and examination of material evidence, comprised in large part of discursive acts.

Ferguson (2001) wrote about the construction of "what it means to be blind." In answer to Hacking's (1999) question (discussed above) of *what* is socially constructed, at this juncture, Ferguson's text responds, "attitudes of the sighted toward the blind." Ferguson described the sighted as perceiving the blind as "less than human" (p. 59). He titled this particular chapter "Pity, Sin, and Myths." Ferguson analyzed the one dozen public beliefs about blindness compiled (at times demonstrably erroneously) by Monbeck (1973), collapsing them into the three themes of the chapter's title. Ferguson traced the first two themes, "pity" to ancient origins, that being the Greek civilization at the time of Plutarch, Plato, and Aristotle, and "sin" to interpretations of religious texts such as the Bible. He explained that in ancient times the blind were "purged from ordinary social interaction with the public" usually through "annihilation" in which blind babies were killed, or sometimes "veneration" in which those blind adults permitted to live were seen as unnatural or perhaps even supernatural (p. 39). Murder was often justified through the association of blindness and sin. Blindness was interpreted as divine punishment for the sins of the individual and/or his/her family.

Ferguson (2001) summarized three of the most pervasive "myths" of blindness. The first is the conceptualization of blindness as "darkness." The association with darkness stirs primeval associations and fears; Jernigan (1965) wrote that darkness is "equated with evil, stupidity, sin, and inferiority" (p. 76). In reality, "more than 80 percent of people with changed vision retain some ability to see" (CNIB, p. 2). And "a totally blind person sees nothing—the absence of any visual sensory stimuli" (Ferguson, p. 45). The second myth is that people's blindness "causes them to be miserable" (Ferguson, p. 46). Throughout the literature (popular, professional, and even much academic) blind people are presented as unhappy and misfortunate. To counter such attitudes, tenBroek (1957) "document[ed] this thesis of the normality of the blind with a random sample of the occupations represented at [the] National Convention [National Federation of the Blind] a year ago" (p. 2). Some of the attendees he listed are: three blind physicists; one blind chemist; two blind full professors; and 13 blind lawyers. tenBroek's (1957) list also serves to contravene the third myth, also described by Scott (1969), namely that the blind are "useless" and "must therefore be dependent on sighted people to survive" (Ferguson, p. 46). Ferguson concluded, "pity, sin and myths about blindness have influenced many to believe that blindness is the worst of all disabilities. Consequently, in the twentieth century, policy makers assumed that blindness was a social problem" (p. 46).

Thus, having constructed blindness as a social problem, the "solution" of professional intervention was enacted. Ferguson (2001) described "the belief that certain social problems are "natural" and that what is needed are solutions that will ease the tragedy of blindness" (p. 81). Ferguson chronicled the tension between the organized blind and the professionals paid to "support" them. The tensions seem to emerge largely through absence—absence of opportunity for the blind to voice their opinions or to take a functional role in the formation of policy and procedure; absence of economic and social liberation in the objectives of the professional organizations; and absence of blind people in positions of influence and leadership. The struggle for self-determination, power, and voice (as described by Shapiro (1993) and others as igniting the formal organization of disabled people) was echoed in the eventual formation of the National Federation of the Blind, even with the historic predominance of the professional organization—the American Foundation for the Blind.

Ferguson (2001) analyzed elements of policy and practice. He described federal legislation and the challenge posed by the organized blind, and analyzed the entrenchment of professional models through establishment of accreditation, and the purposeful exclusion of the blind. He described efforts of the organized blind to confront discrimination and the learning outcomes of political action.

Finally, Ferguson (2001) applied policy archaeology specifically to "the battle for Braille literacy." This section of his text presents a poignant example of the destructive outcomes of "pity" and "myths" such as are described above. Ferguson traced the decline of Braille teaching and usage to an increase in prevalence of blindness beyond the capacity of school boards to provide special education teachers proficient in Braille, and a misapplication of the concept of stigma. Oppressive attitudes toward the blind created a myth that reading a Braille book, thus establishing oneself as identifiably blind, is more stigmatizing than functional illiteracy. Ferguson used an example of a child who was denied Braille instruction because she could read 10 words-per-minute using a text magnifier; a good Braille reader can read 250 words-per-minute, and an advanced reader can achieve 400 words-per-minute.

Blindness: The History of a Mental Image in Western Thought **by Moshe Barasch (2001)**

Barasch (2001) addressed three questions within his text: does the understanding of blindness have a history; what are the interpretations of blindness throughout the "great historical periods" and what brought them about; and how was the blind person imagined (pp. 3-4). Applying Hacking's levels of social constructionism, Barasch's text is "historical." His analysis rests in the past; he did not address the images or interpretations of the present, nor ponder what blindness images of the past mean within a contemporary context. Barasch differentiated between blindness as a phenomenon, and what blindness "means," establishing that it is the latter that is socially constructed. He wrote, "Blindness itself is, of course, a natural condition.... But while blindness as such remains unchanged, our understanding of blindness, our views concerning its "meaning," are matters of culture" (p. 3).

Barasch (2001) began by interpreting blindness within antiquity. Within antiquity, blindness was presented ambiguously, with the linking of seemingly incompatible characterizations. Blindness was seen as punishment (for such crimes as seeing the gods), implicating the blind as guilty.

At the same time (at least in part because some were believed to have been in contact with the gods), they were seen to have supernatural powers. These powers caused them to be held in awe, which was tempered with pity. Barasch explained that these "double natures" instituted "madness" as a characteristic of blindness. The majority of the beliefs of antiquity were "inherited" but refined within the early Christian world (p. 64): the punishment was associated with God's commandments; the gifts were of prophecy; and seeing the gods became "seeing the light," or the "experience of rapture" (p. 65).

While Barasch (2001) interpreted the images of blindness of antiquity as flowing into the early Christian period, he described a metaphorical dam separating off the Middle Ages. The blind were differentiated as "noble" or "common," the first of which dominated the imagery and remained ambiguous (p. 91). The "common" blind were imaged as low-class beggars, who were dishonest and ridiculous. The "noble" blind, or allegorical figures, were imaged as "sinful" and sometimes "disastrous" and at the same time "endowed with majestic dignity" and "believed to hold an irresistible power over man" (p. 64). For example, Barasch described visual depictions of the allegorical synagogue. The synagogue was depicted as a *blind* woman because "its very nature prevented it from seeing and accepting the redemption of Christ" (p. 84). However, its blindness was not depicted as unnatural or gore, but with the "sublime dignity" of a blindfold (p. 87).

Barasch (2001) wrote that the differentiation between high/allegorical and low-class blind continues into the Renaissance, but in an understated manner (particularly of the low-class blind). Barasch considers the paucity of blindness imagery in the Renaissance to be a riddle, considering that vision was so "highly valued" as a "genuine and indispensable organ for the understanding of reality" (p. 115). The blindness images that are revealed make metaphorical blindness prominent. Barasch described the personifications of Fortuna and Cupid, and the image of the blind poet Homer.

Barasch (2001) ended with what he termed Diderot's "disenchantment of blindness" (p. 147). Barasch presented Diderot as a "central figure in the French Enlightenment," who explored the "inner world of the blind" (p. 148). Prior to Diderot's texts, the "overall intellectual upheaval" of the Enlightenment questioned superstition, including beliefs about the blind as demons, and emphasized sensory experience. Diderot's *Lettre* particularly emphasizes the sense of touch. He wrote that in using touch, "the blind person ... is different from the seeing, but not inferior to him" (p. 154). Thus begins the construction of normality.

Analysis of the Leading Journal—*Journal of Visual Impairment and Blindness*

While peer-reviewed papers about blindness appear in a wide variety of academic journals, a search of any digital repository reveals the bulk of literature in the *Journal of Visual Impairment and Blindness* (JVIB). It is also rare to find any text or paper in the blindness domain that does not include some JVIB papers in its reference list. JVIB is self-described as

> the premiere international, interdisciplinary journal of record on blindness and visual impairment that publishes scholarship and information and serves as a forum for the exchange of ideas, airing of controversies, and discussion of issues. JVIB is a monthly publication that includes research articles, as well as shorter pieces of interest to practitioners and extensive news coverage about the field of visual impairment.

JVIB is published through the American Federation for the Blind. With the journal's intellectual domination in the field of blindness, analysis of its current annals reveals both a reflection of contemporary blindness images and the journal editors' construction of what it means to be blind. In other words, through examining the messages conveyed through the journal, a constructionist reveals the dominant meanings. Further, because the journal's discourse has such unparalleled power of circulation in the blindness field, it also serves to influence thinking about blindness.

Of 40 papers in over 700 print pages published in 2005, 36 were reports of original empirical research. The remaining 4 were didactic and/or opinion pieces discussing issues in orientation and mobility (2), depression, and developmental psychology. Of the 36 empirical papers, 23 (64%) reported quantitative or combined quantitative and qualitative research, 8 used qualitative methodology, 4 reported literature reviews and/or meta-analyses and 1 was interpretive. The papers clustered into 10 topic domains. The topic of "rehabilitation" with papers addressing such subjects as vocational rehabilitation, and teaching social interaction skills and oral hygiene was the most frequent, with 10 papers (25%). Two topics tied for second place with respect to frequency with 8 papers each. The "psychology" topic area addressed such constructs as perceived competence, coping, development, and social supports. The "orientation and mobility" (O&M) topic category was elevated in that 6 of the 8 papers came from the October issue, which was a special issue on O&M. There were 4 papers dedicated to "technology" with pieces on such topics as user interfaces and the Internet. Three papers addressed "pathology," taking up sexual abuse, depression, and verbalism. There were 2 papers for each topic of "biomechanics" of vision and "education." The remaining 3 papers were the sole presentations for each topic of "Braille," "policy," and "public attitudes."

Cross analyzing topics with methodology, "rehabilitation" was split evenly, with 5 papers employing purely qualitative approaches, and the other 5 using quantitative or blended quantitative and qualitative approaches. The topics of "orientation and mobility" and "psychology" were largely quantitatively oriented. Five of the 8 O&M papers were quantitative; one was a literature review and the remaining 2 were nonempirical. "Psychology" showed only 1 pure qualitative paper and the sole interpretive piece. The interpretive paper by Ulster and Antle (2005) was titled, "In the Darkness There can be Light: A Family's Adaptation to a Child's Blindness." The paper presents an in-depth case study, examining "assumptions about children's abilities to cope and predominant notions of quality of life."

What does the categorization of the papers published in JVIB in 2005 mean? What are the implications? First, the papers being submitted to JVIB in consideration of publication and/or the papers that pass peer review and thereby appear in the journal are predominantly reporting results of quantitative research. There are questions that are predisposed to quantitative research. For example, knowing the prevalence of experiences of childhood sexual abuse (Kvam, 2005) is important quantitative information that has implications for instituting preventative and treatment practices. However, the near absence of interpretive papers (1/40 2.5%) leaves a huge gap in knowledge. Quantitative research cannot address the societal constructions that perpetuate sexual abuse of blind and visually impaired children, nor can it address what it is like to be an adult who was abused in childhood, or for that matter what goes on in the minds of abusers. We do not hear the voices of the abused or abusers in prevalence studies.

With respect to the topics most frequently represented, it is obvious who has control over what information is circulated in the matrix of blindness and visual impairment. The dominant voice is the professional and/or the professors. The highest proportion of papers addresses rehabilitation; papers are about intervening or changing (doing to) people who are blind or visually impaired. The human services industry is perpetuated and sustained. The dominant discourse reigns supreme. A second industry is sustained and informed on the backs of the blind and visually impaired. Entrenched psychological constructs are empirically validated. Whether coping is a legitimate construct for blind and visually impaired people is not queried. The reader takes it for granted that coping is real—and germane to the experience of blindness. The research quantifies coping by type and degree. The language of numbers effects comparison of people's experiences. Interpretive research would unpack the very notion of coping, examining the historical antecedents and derivation of the construct. Not assuming that blindness is something to cope with, informants would describe what it is like to be blind or visually impaired. Coping may not emerge at all.

Perspectives on Technology

Just as blindness is understood socially, Franklin (1999), McLuhan (1964), and Postman (1992) address technology as a pervasive force in determining the way in which we plan, perceive, and function in our day-to-day lives. Franklin used the metaphor of the world-house. And for her, "technology has built the house in which we all live" (p. 1). The walls, the roof, the rooms, and the furnishings are each of technology, and built by technology. (To use a little irony in the extension of Franklin's metaphor, the house she envisions is the first little pig's straw house, doomed to be blown in by the wolf.)

Franklin (1999) defined "technology" in context. She wrote, "technology involves organization, procedures, symbols, new words, equations, and most of all, a mindset" (p. 3). The aspect of technology she explored with the most passion is technology as practice, or the "ways of doing something" (p. 6). This context moves beyond the way in which we wield tools, or the language used to program the computer, to the way in which we relate to one another, and the "set of socially accepted practices and values" or, in other words, "culture" (p. 6). Franklin recognizes technology as a social phenomenon; how we do things both determines and is determined by the cultural context. Postman (2003) drew a distinction between technology and medium to highlight the social properties of the phenomena. He wrote,

> a technology is to a medium as the brain is to a mind. Like the mind, a medium is a use to which a physical apparatus is put. A technology becomes a medium as it is given a place in a particular social setting, as it insinuates itself into economic and political contexts. (p. 184)

Franklin (1999) traced the shift from holistic to prescriptive technologies (defined not as *what* but *how*). She likened the former to a craft whereby the artist has creative license, makes judgements and decisions throughout the process, and has the satisfaction of the final product. The latter is best visualized as division of labor, whereby each person is responsible for steps in the entire project (whether product, policy, or economy). The project is preplanned and overseen. Holistic technologies foster growth. Growth is dynamic and organic in that it "occurs" rather than being "made." Prescriptive technologies are based on a production model, and production can be planned, controlled, and measured. Franklin believes that education is wrongfully structured in accordance with a production model. As evidence, she cited the schedule, the quantification of success in marks and the products of the schooling put out by specialized campuses.

What are the cultural consequences of the dominance of prescriptive technological models? Franklin sees the contemporary disregard for context including the environment as a consequence. She also links a decline in personal responsibility and judgement due to the removed necessity within shared and overseen projects, to the demoted importance of value-based decisions. She wrote,

> while we should not forget that these prescriptive technologies are often exceedingly effective and efficient, they come with an enormous social mortgage. The mortgage means that we live in a culture of compliance, that we are ever more conditioned to accept orthodoxy as normal, and to accept that there is only one way of doing "it." (p. 17)

What are the implications of a culture shaped by the discourse of prescriptive technological processes on *blind* citizens? First, the "culture of compliance" means compliance not only with societal rules and regulations, but with normality. Normality does not recognize the actual frailty and diversity of humans, but is instead defined by those with highest status—White, able-bodied, and some would say, male (Marks, 1999). As revealed by the social constructionist analyses within the matrix of blindness reviewed above, blind people are stigmatized, or to use another of Goffman's (1963) terms, "discredited." They are stigmatized by misinterpretations of what lack of vision means for life functioning, and by misassociations with other stigmatizing conditions of wrongfully attributed emotional dysfunction.

In his assertion that "the medium is the message" McLuhan (1964) explained that one of the consequences of literacy was the expectation of the homogenized man. He wrote, "literate man is quite inclined to see others who cannot conform as somewhat pathetic" (p. 31). He wrote specifically of the technological/discursive exclusion of the blind in his statement, "unaware of our typographic cultural bias, our testers [psychologists assessing intelligence quotients] assume that uniform and continuous habits are a sign of intelligence, thus eliminating the ear man and the tactile man" (pp. 31-32). Batron, a blind technology specialist, stated, "blind learners are not necessarily impeded because they can't see the screen. They will just have to navigate with their ears rather than their eyes" (Batron & Smith, personal correspondence, 2002).

The second discursive construction in the narrative of prescriptive technology as it affects the blind is an impression that the mighty technology has left the blind behind. Franklin (1999) wrote that we seem to have "an inherent trust in machines and devices" (p. 25). We position people as the "source" of problems, and technology as the "solution" (p. 25). With all of the potential for genetic screening and engineering, and the advertisements for reparative surgery including bringing people's vision to 20/20, those with diseases such as diabetic retinopathy cannot have their vision restored through technology. Is this perhaps an embarrassment or a blow to our faith in the power of technology?

Third, as long as the assigned roles are efficiently carried out, the individuals within a prescriptive enterprise are independent. The sense of community is secondary to personal accomplishment and contribution. Dependence, such as for orientation or navigation, is devalued and considered a failing (Dossa, 1990).

Like Franklin (1999), Seelman (2001) examined the impact of technology on our social lives. However, Seelman's text differs from Franklin's in three important ways. First, Seelman focused the context of her inquiry to the disabled. Second, whereas Franklin asserted that science is not the "mother" of technology, and that instead they are two overlapping "fields of endeavour" (p. 30), Seelman married the two and presented their discourses as inseparable. Third, Franklin focused on the aspect of technology that addresses "how we do things" whereas Seelman focused on "what is produced" and "how."

Seelman (2001) positioned adaptive technology [Seelman used the term *assistive* technology—adaptive technology will be used in this text for consistency] at the intersection between science and technology and social models of disability. She defined adaptive technology as, "any item, piece of equipment, or product system—off the shelf, customized, or modified —that is used to increase, maintain, or improve functional capacities of disabled individuals" (p. 664). She used examples of adaptive technology such as wheelchairs, prosthetics, and built-in accessibility features of computer operating systems.

Seelman (2001) addressed seven problems positioned at the intersection of science, technology, and disability. First, technology has not been consistently recognized as subject to social values and priorities, and as such, inquiry has not rigorously been applied to the social consequences. She gave the example of cochlear implants that Shapiro (1993) described as "cultural murder" (p. 223). Second, technological decision making has been "expert-driven" (professionals). Disabled people are rarely invited to the table. Further, the few tables at which they sit are usually advisory without the power to decide policy. Third, the outcomes of technological application to disability are unimpressive. Seelman described the "adaptive technology marketplace" as "fragmented, small, and weak" (p. 670). Fourth, applications of technology for the disabled are slotted into a narrow category that leads to confining solutions and further entrenchment of the disabled into perceived roles of illness and financial dependence—health and benefits. Fifth, the disabled are rarely liberated from roles as research subjects to the role of researcher. Sixth, priorities have been decided by researcher interest and funding availability rather than motivated by emancipatory objectives. Finally, research on adaptive devices has been primarily conducted in clinical settings (rather than tested in the "real world") and without inquiring into the lived experience of the users.

Seelman's (2001) analysis of the contemporary U.S. problems in disabled applications of science and technology is informed in part by a three-part framework of post-World War II scientific mind-sets (pp. 674-685). The first is roughly described as spanning from 1945-1965 and is titled "The Age of the Scientist and the Professional." Adaptive technology was almost exclusively within the medical domain, including prosthetics and orthotics. Seelman wrote, "early identification of adaptive technology within medical technology may be the basis of seemingly intractable perception within policy that links the technology needs of disabled people with the health domain" (p. 675). The next stage (1966-1980) is described as "the age of dissent." In some instances, adaptive technology became more broadly defined as "aids and devices" and the vocabulary of "normalization, full participation, and quality of life" was entered into debates (p. 678). The concept of "universal design of the social environment" was also introduced (p. 678). The next stage (1981-1999) takes us closest to the present, and is described as "a period of economic hegemony" (p. 680). Seelman wrote that this period was characterized by "the alignment of research and development with economic objectives" (p. 680).

NFB's Position on Technology

The National Federation of the Blind (NFB)'s position on technology is published as an introduction to the goals of the National Research and Training Institute for the Blind in *The Braille Monitor* (2000, February). The NFB's discursive construction of educational technology might be positioned as what Boshier and Mun Onn (2000) call techno-structuralism. The NFB believes that technology can enhance the educational experiences of blind learners, if applied equitably and with attention to issues of power.

> Technology is a critical element in both education and employment opportunities today and will be even more so in the future, for the blind just as for the general public. Advances in speech, Braille, and large-print access technology lead some to assume that the blind now have or soon will have access to nearly all of what technology has to offer.... Unfortunately, due to the widespread obsession with visual design in technology, the shortage of good technology training, the cost of equipment, and the rapid advancements of technology applications, blind people now face the dismaying prospect of being left out if nonvisual [sic.] access is not continually updated and improved. This means that advances in software and hardware must include design that allows nonvisual access. (p. 5)

The NFB asserts the importance of nonvisual design. This is in keeping with what disability studies scholars call "universal design." Marks (1999) explained that universal design is "concerned to produce a 'flexible architecture' based on structures which are 'demountable, reasonable, multi-functional and changeable over time' " (p. 86). Within the context of educational technology, as a rule, today's computer applications are designed for technically proficient, 20-to-30-year-olds with no sensory or mobility impairments. Marks described this as the "ableist" design of the "built" environment. The expectation is that so-called "deviants" from this profile, not be resistant to adaptive devices, accommodations or adaptations. Yet, the NFB's statement does not advocate advances in adaptive technology or accommodations and adaptations to the delivery of a standard course designed with only the "able-bodied" student in mind. The NFB is advocating for a universal design.

Conclusion

Asch (1995) began her invitational entry on "visual impairment" for the *Encyclopedia of Social Work* with her presentation of what she heard through a 1994 public radio broadcast that she described as "vividly captur[ing] the prevailing images of blindness" (p. 636). Her description of this image warrants an extended quotation.

> The story described a fifty-three-year-old Mexican immigrant to the United States whose work as an accordionist and singer in the New York City subways "amazes and entertains even the most cynical riders." According to the NPR reporter, "What made this so incredible was that the musician was blind. But there he was, moving slowly through the swaying and speeding car, never missing a beat in the music, never losing his balance." She reported that nickels, dimes, quarters, and dollar bills began "to fill the white plastic cup taped to his accordion...." She closed the program by saying that the man "must have an angel looking over him." (pp. 636-637)

These contemporary images are consistent with those unearthed by Scott (1969), Ferguson (2001), and most remarkably, with those found in antiquity by Barasch (2001). The images are not counter-acted by the papers currently reaching circulation through the *Journal of Visual Impairment and Blindness* (JVIB). Images of the blind cluster into three categories of humanity. Images of the blind as *subhuman* or demonic were somewhat obliterated through rejection of superstition in the Enlightenment (Barasch), but can still be detected in hesitation to approach the blind, "cynicism" and "fear of the unknown." The construction of the blind as *low-human* continues to dominate, as depicted as pitiable and somewhat pathetic, and defined in the role of beggar, relegated to a life of poverty, and as the dominance of papers in JVIB indicates—in need of rehabilitation. Even in the inherited differentiation between the low- and high-class blind, the "high-class" blind are underrepresented in postsecondary education (U.S. Department of Education, 1999; Walker, 1994) and a "missing factor" in science and technology policy (Seelman, 2001). Finally, the blind are imaged as *superhuman*. Asch's (1995) described man is the "blind singer-seer" imaged in antiquity (Barasch, p. 44). In the secular version of divine vision, the man is gifted with the compensatory ability to keep his balance in the moving subway. Nonsecular, is the image of his companionship with the watching angels.

In considering the implications of these images on application of educational technologies, we must also be cognizant of the constructed triad of images of technology. Replacing the above word "human" with "moral," as we have seen, authors such as Franklin (1999) and Postman (1992) image technology as a subversive force or *submoral*. *Low-moral* images include technology as a poor substitute for human sensory experience, transforming that experience to one of isolation and disembodiment (e.g., Dreyfus, 2001). Finally, advocates for "bringing the disabled to the table of technology" create images of *supermorality*, stating that technology will "level the playing field" (Coombs & Banks, 2000).

Remarkably absent in antiquity and today is the experiential, the reflexive—the voice of the blind—particularly the voice of those who have reclaimed the idea of blindness, obliterating what French and Swain (2001) label "epistemic invalidation" (p. 738) and what others have labeled "phenomenological doubt." Even Diderot's *Lettre* "disenchanting blindness" was constructed with an imaginary informant. Awareness of the images of blindness and of technology and their overlap can facilitate better empirical research into the lived experience of the blind, but the imperative to systematically ask blind people themselves what it is like to use technologies remains unanswered.

CHAPTER 3

INTERPRETING RESEARCH

Generally defined, research is the intentional pursuit of discovery, or in other words, a process designed to answer questions. There is much to be said for quantitative research when what one needs is a summary or a prediction. For example, if one wants to know whether children in one school district are scoring higher in their annual examinations than in another district, the proportion of blind children per area, or the likelihood that blind applicants will be accepted into postsecondary institutions, only quantitative research can answer these questions. Many impressive and famous outcomes have derived from quantitative research. For example, the world celebrated research's contribution to ending the polio plague and preventing small pox. As depicted in Deborah's story in chapter 5, medical research into Retinoblastoma between Deborah's childhood and her daughter's birth meant that Deborah is totally blind whereas her daughter, born with the same condition, requires only corrective lenses and is not even legally blind.

Researchers have tried to replicate the same type of success experienced in the domains that lend themselves to quantitative research, to questions of human relationships and perceptions. To their dismay, it does not work. It usually yields trivial, meaningless, results. Postman (1993) wrote that the contribution of human sciences is in telling the story in new and compelling ways that motivate people to action, not in creating new knowledge.

Seeing Beyond Blindness, 39–43

When our questions concern culture or relationships between people, then our research supersedes the type of information that the symbols of numbers as used in quantitative research can communicate. Language, culture, how people present themselves, who they choose to present and power imbalances all come into play when inquiring into the lives of humans. The concepts of postmodernism, discourse, reflexivity, and social identity are fundamental to social science research.

Postmodernism

Postmodernism defies definition, because postmodernists do not believe in fixing complex constructions into denotative definitions. Postmodernism cannot be reined-in because there is no one meaning; the very nature of post-modernism is multiple voices, multiple meanings. There are also no pure postmodernists because theorists informed by such conceptualizations have witnessed the fall-out of conversion to one or another trends, ideologies, or metanarratives, and are thereby not "true believers" in anything including postmodernism. For all of these reasons, postmodernism is one of the most challenging terms to write about in plain language.

Insofar as a postmodernist perspective informs both reflections on vision in contemporary Middle America and the interpretive approach to the research elaborated in the following chapters, it is important to initiate some shared understanding of postmodern thinking. As a face reading of the term suggests, postmodernism can only be understood as a reaction to modernism. The hallmark of modernism is the grand narrative of science and scientific thinking. Science, with its systematic method to acquire understanding, allowed *man*kind to represent, measure, manipulate, and often master the world around him. Through practicing science, man travelled to the moon, inoculated against many different strands of disease, and created nuclear weapons. Science and those engaged in its pure practice were elevated above other mortals. Their voices became privileged and *other* voices became silenced or muted. Science became reified and deified casting religion as *blind* faith. Science became *the* route to knowledge and it became heresy (in a Godless time) to suggest that there were other ways of knowing. For one example, consider the reaction to the privilege of evolution over creationism.

Postmodernism throws everything into question; it leaves no stone unturned. In postmodern times, there is no adherence to the privileged authority. The king's voice is no more privileged than the pauper (and the sighted no more than the blind) and knowledge is situated. In order to interlocute regarding experience, one must engage within the context of the other. Further, the concept of *other* is held suspect. While the privileged voice is made to be the center of the revered normal curve, in world prevalence, white European-derived, able-bodied, educated, mostly-males are outliers. In modern times their voice is dominant. The insidious practice of comparing and ranking people by the normal curve is made salient and toppled. Of what significance is the low-incidence categorization of blindness? Postmodernist researchers seek the contrasting voices. *Others* are urged to speak for themselves, not veiled through the agendas of the dominant. Researchers, whether quantitative or qualitative, are urged to challenge the power dynamic that allows them to determine the questions, represent the experience of others, and then reap the reward. Post-modern research does not exist in a vacuum to be applied as it will by others. Research is an ethical pursuit, enacting change throughout the process even if the researchers seek only to observe.

Science is understood as a discourse, not *the* route to understanding and mastering an external reality. Further, there is no external reality *out-there* to be represented and indelibly communicated. *Seeing* is representing something *as* something, implicating interpretation, symbolic construction, and the problem of shared communication within multiple contexts. Scientific representation is just as subject to interpretation as any other discipline. The scientists, developing and designing their experiments, interpreting the results, and then making them salient through communication, do so within a time and place context.

Discourse

Foucault (1972) presented discursive formations, recognizing the importance of language in shaping interpretations and meanings of our social world. R. J. Ferguson (2001) used policy archaeology, an application of Foucault's archaeology, to examine social and educational experiences of the blind. The webs of educational phenomena are spun from language, and more specifically of discourse. Discourse includes the meanings or conceptions of reality, often held as truths or unexamined assumptions shared and communicated by a group of people. Spradley (1979) wrote, "language is more than a means of communication about reality: it is a tool for constructing reality" (p. 17). In other words, the body of literature (including scholarly peer-reviewed publications, marketing documents, and WWW pages) serves to describe phenomena in fields such as educational technology, and at the same time, it constructs or shapes the way in which that reality is interpreted, and the developments that follow. With respect to distance education research, test scores, bulletin board transcripts, and course evaluations are not sufficient indicators of what it is like to be a blind online learner. The phenomenological experience of the learners necessitates research through the informants' depictions. Learners need to tell their own stories. What they choose to say and leave out of their descriptions of online learning both reflect and construct that experience.

Such notions of reflexivity are intertwined in complex ways with notions of technological determinism, leading us to ask whether technology is just a tool or whether the prevalent technologies determine our interpretations of our social reality including the applications to which we put those technologies. McLuhan (1964) wrote that the medium is the message. Franklin (1999) described our culture as living in the house that technology has built. With respect to distance education research, whether online learning has the capacity to open-up participation of blind adults in post-secondary education is one important consideration. The social ramifications of adoption of online technologies need also be considered. In pursuing what it is like to be a blind online learner, the experience necessitates pursuance beyond the functionality of the tools to the social consequences of their adoption.

Reflexivity

Reflexivity necessitates mindful attention to the power of language to both reflect and construct meaning. Alvesson and Sköldberg (2000) explained,

> Reflection (reflexivity) is thus above all a question of recognizing fully the notoriously ambivalent relation of a researcher's text to the realities studied. Reflection means interpreting one's own perspectives from other perspectives, and turning a self-critical eye onto one's own authority as interpreter and author. (p. vii)

Thus in producing a literature review, it is important to recognize the impact of individual pieces, their meaning within the context of the other topical writings, and the meaning constructed through their interweaving. In considering the interview transcripts it is important to consider the relationship between the researcher and the informants in the telling and the writing-up of the stories. In writing the interpretive chapters, it is important to acknowledge the meeting of the informants' stories with the social history of the author.

Social Identity

The fourth philosophical perspective prevalent to human science research concerns social identity. Goffman's (1959) analysis of the means by which people present themselves in metaphorical social performances applies beyond "live" interactions, including the significance of written literature to the understanding of ourselves and others. The literature is produced and interpreted within a social context. Goffman's (1963) theories are particularly relevant to research into the blindness domain, in that he applied social presentation specifically to those residing outside the normative or acceptable social realm—the stigmatized. The literature on the educational experiences of the blind must be interpreted in a context in which the learners have been restricted by the social construction of "what it means to be blind" (Ferguson, 2001, p. 38).

Hermeneutic phenomenological research, influenced by seminal writers such as Gadamer (1960), Habermas (1972), and Heidegger (1977) inquires into lived experience (van Manen, 1997). Within the research presented in the pages to follow, hermeneutic phenomenological inquiry facilitates asking what it is like to be a blind learner. Phenomenology challenges researchers to describe experience. Moustakas (1994) provided the rationale and imperative of phenomenological research,

> The only way I can truly come to know things and people is to go out to them, to return again and again to them, to immerse myself completely in what is there before me, look, see, listen, hear, touch, from many angles and perspectives and vantage points, each time freshly so that there will be continual openings and learnings that will connect with each other and with prior perceptions, understandings, and future possibilities. In other words, I must immerse myself totally and completely in my world, take in what is offered without bias or prejudgment. I must pause and consider what my own life is and means, in conscious awareness, in thought, in reflections. (p. 65)

The following chapters explicate one such deep inquiry. Research into *Blind Online Learners* is presented and annotated not only to explicate the results, but to inquire into the process of conducting interpretive research.

CHAPTER 4

RESEARCH EXEMPLIFIED

Blind Online Learners

OVERVIEW

The following research is used as an example of interpretive research in the field of blindness. Discussion is situated by this example; the flood gates open and close to fluctuate between general discussion of interpretive research and the specific examples generated by this instance of inquiry. Interactive interviews were conducted with five adults who are totally blind and two adults who have low vision and have been labeled legally blind to inquire: (a) what it is like to be a blind online learner, (b) what comprise the best online learning design characteristics, and (c) what impact is yielded by blind adults studying online. Each informant was the only blind learner amongst sighted colleagues. Six of the respondents use JAWS screen reading software and one uses ZoomText screen enlarging software. Experiences ranged from graduating from a master's degree in which most of the courses were delivered online to withdrawing from an online cooking class due to the frustrating interface and what was perceived as the unsuitable match of content and delivery. Reflexive analysis involved interaction with the empirical material, interpretation, criti-

Seeing Beyond Blindness, 45–60

cal theoretical reflection, and discourse analysis. Five of the seven participants evaluated online learning positively. One of the two participants evaluating online learning negatively was the woman who withdrew from the cooking course. The other learner enrolled in a noninteractive course. The four main research findings are: (a) online learning is possible, convenient and prodigious for blind adults; (b) three essential characteristics of online learning are simplicity, interactivity, and accessibility; (c) blind learners require access to and working knowledge of adaptive technologies as well as either a high level of technological proficiency or regular access to human supports; and (d) course characteristics designed to benefit blind learners improve online learning for all students.

Research Benefits

Research is a time and energy consuming pursuit on the part of both the researcher and the participants. It is important that we move beyond the ethic of "do no harm" to the consideration of what benefit might derive from our pursuits. For the researcher, the perceived benefits of this particular research were to increase understanding of interpretive methods and to become a better online instructor and course designer. For the research participants, the researcher was available to answer questions about blind online learning. In addition, participants may receive indirect benefit through post-secondary institutional application of research findings in terms of how to make online learning accessible. For the research community, the study may provide insight and application into best practices in online learning, thus enhancing academic distribution of knowledge. Finally, for society at large, a better understanding of online learning may lead to more effective postsecondary education.

Methodology

More and more, research in the interpretive domain does not choose a particular methodology such as pure hermeneutics, grounded theory, or ethnography. Instead, research borrows from these various approaches, drawing from the strengths and philosophical undergirdings of each. Likewise, this particular research did not use a unitary methodology. Kincheloe and Berry (2004) described this approach to research as a bricolage. Aspland (1999) described her journey as the "evolution of a methodological pastiche" explaining that it is a "work of methodological art whereby perceived incongruent forms come together seemingly in opposition, yet ultimately creat[ing] a research framework that is cohesive" (p. 106).

Aspland's (1999) incorporation of phenomenology, feminist research, and critical ethnography resonated with the approach of this inquiry. Informed by phenomenological hermeneutics, this research sought to represent the students' experiences and autobiographical interpretations of being in online education. Research in the domain of disability studies resonates with feminist research. Both acknowledge and honor the experiences of those with minority status, who may have been stigmatized, oppressed, and disempowered. Both recognize the social construction of definitions and roles. Both seek participatory frameworks. Informed by critical ethnography, the researcher was a participant observer, sharing experiences as a doctoral student and online instructor to open-up dialogue representing and reflexively constructing the research and the learning experience.

The Origins of Research

Empirical research is driven by curiosity. The researcher wants to know something. Often observations are made that are counterintuitive and leave one wondering why, or suspicions beg to be confirmed. Also frequently, one's reading reveals a gap in the literature that can only be addressed empirically. This was the case with this research. There was a paucity of literature at the intersection of online learning and disability and even less specific to blind online learners.

The Literature

There are a small number of publications positioned at the overlap between distance education and disability. Of those, very few are research—and the source publications are largely conferences and journals within the field of disability studies rather than in mainstream educational technology. In a comprehensive search, I found 67 publications released between 2000 and 2006 that were situated at the intersection of distance education and disability. In this review, "publications" are defined as journal articles, government and newspaper reports, and full-article conference proceedings. Proceedings from the 2000-2006 Technology and Persons with Disabilities Conferences through California State University Northridge's (CSUN) Center on Disabilities comprise 39% of the publications. The number of CSUN presentations in the topic stream of distance education shows a steady rate of increase until 2003, with two presentations in 2000, three in 2001, nine in 2002, and eleven in 2003. In 2004 and 2005, presentation in this stream declined with two and three respectively. Analysis of the conference proceedings enabled me to conduct a more lucrative search, expanding key search terms to contemporary constructs, such as "universal design," "assistive technologies," and "accessible learning;" conference presenters (e.g. Burgstahler) as publishing authors; and organizations' Web sites with links, such as Equal Access to Software and Information.

Of the 67 publications, 27 (40%) are didactic. They present guidelines and how-to information in regard to a single or combination of topics including accessibility, communication tools, instructional design, pedagogy, policy, teaching strategies, and universal design. The next highest category of publications (18, or 27%) is description of vendor products and/or educational programs (including postsecondary institutions and private industry). The lowest category can best be classified as editorials or opinion pieces at five articles (7%).

Seventeen articles (25%) can be counted as research. Even this small amount of research is a recent phenomenon; 12 of the articles have 2003 to 2006 as their publication dates. The total is amplified in that 11 of the 17 articles are written by 4 first-authors (Fichten, 4; Kim-Rupnow, 2; Kinash, 3; and Richardson, 2). Further, 2 of the Kinash articles and 2 of the Fichten articles are multiple depictions of the same research. To date there is a small body of researchers producing a small body of research largely in their fields of concentration.

The main paper begging the facilitation of this particular research was Kim-Rupnow, Dowrick, and Burke's (2001—perhaps one day in the future when distributed education using digital media has had a much longer history—considered *seminal* at the intersection of disability and online learning. Not only is their paper one of a mere handful of research initiatives in this area, but the authors have sought to establish a foundation, or a platform from which to launch more in-depth inquiry. The question driving their analysis of the literature was, "Do the increase in distance education programs and use of advanced technology indicate better access and better outcomes in higher education for persons with disabilities?" (p. 25). They answered positively, yet inconclusively due to the paucity of research. Using electronic databases of published journal articles and manual searches of the table of contents of distance education journals, the authors derived ten articles. Each of the 10 articles includes information about postsecondary students with disabilities enrolled in distance education courses. Most of the articles were written from the perspective of the postsecondary institution and include very brief descriptions of one or two students with disabilities.

Although not explicitly differentiated by the authors, some of the emerging themes resonate with issues for all postsecondary distance education support systems regardless of whether or not the respective students are disabled whereas the others appear to be the contribution of technological advances for supporting postsecondary students with disabilities at a distance. The more general themes are: (a) student prior experience with computers (this emerged as a common characteristic of the students depicted in the literature), (b) university programs delivering online learning using a combination of several technologies (including multimedia and some interactive platforms) and, (c) varied use of synchronous and/or asynchronous communication tools for collaboration. The themes closely related to disabilities are: (a) availability of technical assistance to facilitate content accessibility (examples include transcribed text and interpretation), (b) formats that are not effectively translated by text readers (such as tables and graphics), (c) university supports extended to disabled students (such as access to home computers and assistive devices) and, (d) existence of an individualized education (and/or accommodation) plan for learners with disabilities.

One of the overarching themes in the small amount of literature situated at the intersection of online learning and disability is that the theory and practical application of research with disabled learners has the potential to enhance the pedagogical potential of online learning for all postsecondary students. Application of accessible online learning provides "electronic curb-cuts" for all learners. Cook and Gladhart's (2002) paper stated and supported this proposition explicitly. However, its mainstream reception might be limited by its location in the niche readership of the journal of *Information Technology and Disabilities*. Kim-Rupnow, Dowrick, and Burke's (2001) paper did not address universal design and the serendipitous results of making online learning accessible to people with disabilities. However, its positioning in the *American Journal of Distance Education* may, in any case, raise awareness of the existence and needs of online learners with disabilities. Those applying the accessibility modifications may serendipitously reap the benefits of improved usability for all learners.

To use the colloquial, one of the pivotal issues in online learning can be categorized as a "chicken and egg" debate. Is online learning an "authentic educational technology" wherein problems in higher learning were identified, and online learning was developed as the solution? Or, did a technological imperative prompt the adoption of online learning? (Clark & Estes, 1999). In the latter case, some would suggest that online learning is serendipitous. The learner needs were rasping against the university systems creating a rash of discontent. Online learning tends to draw learners who are older, employed full-time, married, and often female

(Thompson, 1998). Perhaps the pedagogical, geographical, and multimedia flexibility of online learning can rectify the problems and match the needs of the contemporary student. Online learning is advertised as facilitating anytime, anywhere learning, and with more attention to accessibility issues, has the potential to also suit the needs of any learner.

At least one subset of the student population—disabled adults—do not seem to be well-served by the postsecondary system. Students with disabilities are underrepresented. The percentage of 1995-96 U.S.A. undergraduates who reported a disability was estimated at 6% (U.S. National Center for Education Statistics, 1999). The low proportion of postsecondary students with disabilities is tragic considering that graduates appear to be hired into positions equivalent to their nondisabled colleagues (U.S. National Center for Education Statistics, 1999). What little literature that exists informing what it is like to be a disabled post-secondary student indicates an unwillingness to make courses accessible to disabled learners, and/or to accommodate particular support needs (when these emerge).

It has been suggested that online learning is a positive initiative for postsecondary students with disabilities. Online learning has the potential to be accessible in space, time, and format. Students are not required to travel to a campus and cope with impediments to mobility. Much of online learning is asynchronous, and can therefore be accessed at hours that fit into full-lives. Because the information is digital, it can be "pulled" in the format that best suits the learner, whether that be audio, visual, or a combination.

A techno-structuralist view of online learning, balances the optimism of the potential of online learning to meet the needs of students with disabilities, with provisos and cautions (McGrane, 2000). The question remains as to whether the dominance of visual interfaces can and will be balanced with auditory options. There is also question as to whether online learning will become a new type of segregated education, denying blind learners an avenue of social interaction, and missing an opportunity for public stereotypes and stigma to be confronted and challenged through face-to-face interaction with blind student colleagues.

The questions posed by Kim-Rupnow, Dowrick, and Burke in 2001 remain unresolved. These questions need to be posed once again, urging further study: (a) is the prevalence of online learning increasing postsecondary access to students with disabilities; (b) what services are most important in supporting postsecondary online learners; (c) what are the long-term outcomes of online learners with disabilities; and (d) what "standard accommodations" and innovations "especially encourage diverse learners" (p. 37)? To these, a review of the literature adds the questions: (a) what is it like to be an online learner with disabilities; and (b) how can we promote universal design of the online environment, with particular emphasis on complimenting the visual with the auditory interface? The answer to the latter question may lie in the intersection of the promise afforded by online learning technology, and the needs of learners and teachers with disabilities, recognizing the potential of multimedia to support multiple learning styles and needs.

The Research Questions

The gaps emerging from the literature were clustered into three questions: (a) what is it like to be a blind online learner, (b) what are the best design characteristics of online learning, and (c) what is the impact of blind learners studying online. The first research question precedes the other two. The personal experiences and way in which informants perceive these experiences informs an inquiry into whether or not online learning is a prodigious educational venture for blind adults. Kim-Rupnow, Dowrick, and Burke's (2001) questions are represented in the latter two research questions. Querying the best design of online learning involves asking what services and supports are necessary and whether innovation and accommodation are required beyond the design of the courses for the sighted learners. The additional question emerging beyond Kim-Rupnow et al.'s interpretation involves the best design of online learning. Is it possible and advantageous to design online courses and programs such that they are accessible by all learners without the addition of specialized services, supports, innovations, and accommodations? Informants were asked how the courses were structured, whether they used learning moderation systems, and what type. They were also asked to describe and demonstrate the use of adaptive technologies and the compatibility between such technologies and courseware. It was queried whether the students' programs were entirely online, or whether they experienced a blended model whereby some courses were online and others face-to-face. We also discussed the degree of interactivity and the tasks facilitating interaction, and the nature of assignments. Informants were asked to describe and comment on their experience of communication tools and courseware used to present learning modules.

The third question regarding the impact of online learning was intentionally worded ambiguously. Not specifying the object of the impact enabled the research to remain open. The impact might be on the disabled students themselves, on their student colleagues, on the instructor, on the course content and design, on the university administrative structure and information technology systems, or some combination. While the conversation remained open, analysis queried such questions as whether blind students are accessing post-secondary education through online programs and what comprise the outcomes of enrolment in online programs. In other words, are blind students applying, being admitted, and graduating from online postsecondary programs? Are they fulfilling their pre-enrollment goals? For example, if the program goal is to secure employment, are they securing employment upon graduation?

The Research Method

In order to explore these questions, seven online learners who are blind were interviewed. The research participants were recruited through multiple public postings, drawing adults who are studying or have graduated from a variety of American and Canadian postsecondary institutions and private industry. The individual stories of the seven informants are presented. Each story addresses what it was like for that individual to be a blind online learner, what design characteristics worked and did not work for him/her personally, and what impact he/she perceived from the experience on him or herself and for those involved in the experience through association such as fellow students, instructors, and university administrators. Next, the experiences were considered in combination. What can the commonalities and differences of the experiences of seven individuals reflect regarding online learning for blind and sighted students in general? The phenomenological experience of online learning was analyzed through a series of grids. The grids enabled investigation into questions such as—of the seven informants, are the learners who experienced online learning as accessible more likely to evaluate the experience as positive than learners who experienced online learning as inaccessible? Best practices were analyzed in terms of how the experiences of the seven informants resonate with Coombs and Banks' (2000) tips for the design and instruction of online learning. The impact was analyzed both inductively and deductively. Participants' interpretations of impact emerged unprovoked within their descriptions of their experiences. Themes of impact also emerged within the literature. Questions addressing these issues of impact were posed to the respondents. Analysis compared the interpretation presented by the literature with that shared by the respondents.

The next layer is a critical theoretical approach to the interview data. This research is grounded in social constructionism. Attitudes toward blindness, the way in which blind people are treated, the design of online learning and ways in which blind students experience online learning are constructed by American and Canadian culture. There are political underpinnings to online learning within educational institutions and to the education of blind adults. The stories of the seven online learners were revisited through this critical theoretical lenses. Three questions were posed: (1) What bias was introduced by interpreting blind online learning through the perspectives of these particular seven adults? (2) How does the American and Canadian social construction of blindness impact perceptions of what it is like to be a blind online learner? (3) What impact does technological imperative have on practices in online learning?

Applying discourse analysis, the next layer of inquiry derived out of the perspective that language both reflects and constructs experience. The experience of online learning is storied by the participants. Elements of the experience become salient even for the participants through the words that they use to describe the events and circumstances. Analysis was conducted through considering the relationship between the interviewer and the respondents and how this interlocution impacts the stories that are told. Two open pieces of dialogue were considered. Informants were asked what it is like to be a blind online learner and to tell whatever they would like to share about themselves personally. Analysis involved interpreting what themes emerged and in what order.

Recruitment

The participants in this research were selected based on the criteria of: (a) adult age status, (b) legal blindness as self-reported, (c) computer access through the use of adaptive technologies, (d) previous enrollment in one or more online courses, and (e) willingness to participate in digitally videotaped interviews that will become public domain. A triangulation of recruitment strategies resulted in what appeared to be a breadth of information dissemination. An invitation to participate was posted in publicly distributed media of the Professional Development and Research Institute on Blindness at Louisiana Tech University and the Louisiana Center for the Blind. A call for participation was posted on two LISTSERVs of The National Federation of the Blind, and on a national LISTSERV of the Canadian National Institute for the Blind (CNIB). The conference organizers of the Pacific Rim Conference in Honolulu in February 2003, and the CSUN Conference in Los Angeles in March 2003 were asked to distribute information regarding the research to potential participants. An invitation to participate was included in all correspondence with my colleagues who are blind. Instructors from Equal Access to Software and Information (EASI) were asked to distribute information to their course graduates. Faculty from universities advertising programs with disability-specific content and/or the enrollment of students with disabilities were asked to distribute information to their students and graduates. The multiple means of distributing information resulted in word-of-mouth dissemination. Three of the research participants were contacted by multiple sources. Bernice, for example, was contacted by EASI, by representatives of CNIB, and by faculty of her local university.

Quantitative researchers frequently have the comfort of equations used to generate a satisfactory number of research participants. Interpretive researchers have to make more difficult decisions about when saturation of information is reached. In other words, when are novel, intriguing and challenging points of views or thematic perspectives no longer introduced by the addition of new participants? Both have to contend with the instrumental realities of budgets and travel restrictions.

In addition to the seven research participants, interest in participating was received from a number of other individuals. Eight of these individuals were interested in online learning, but had not yet enrolled in a course. Two met the criteria and were scheduled for interviews, but circumstances resulted in cancellation. Seven others also met the criteria, but were located beyond the means of a research travel budget that already included long-distance travel to three locations. These seven correspondences were received from Binghamton, Cleveland, Kingston, San Carlos, South Carolina, Toronto, and Winnipeg. The seven interviewed participants fulfilled thematic saturation as will be elaborated below.

The Interview Process

Between January and March 2003, seven blind adults who use adaptive technologies to access the computer and who have previously enrolled-in (and not necessarily completed) one or more online courses were individually interviewed. The initial interviews were held at five geographical locations: urban central Alberta; rural central Alberta; the proximity of the Pacific Rim Conference on Disability in Honolulu, Hawaii; the proximity of the CSUN Conference on Disability and Technology in Los Angeles, California; and two sites in lower mainland, British Columbia.

Interactive Initial Interviews

Throughout the literature (Berg, 1995; Marshall & Rossman, 1989; Merriam, 1998; Neuman, 1997) interviews typically fall into the qualitative research field and are most commonly defined as conversations with the purpose of gathering information. Berg used a dramaturgical metaphor for depicting the research interview, framing it in terms of an encounter, or a face-to-face interactive social performance (p. 30). The interview is like a play in that the participants adopt the roles of interviewer and interviewee and these roles have shared social meanings and unspoken rules. Further, the content of the interview reflects reality, but is like the script of a play in that the lines do not happen spontaneously in the midst of action. Distinguishing qualitative interviews from natural conversation, Berg asserted that the research interview "is not a natural communication exchange" (p. 43). He used the example of the way in which participants in natural conversation develop avoidance strategies and send cues usually respected by the others in the dialogue. However, within research, the interviewer must encourage open communication and discourage such avoidance. While questions and/or topics are pre-established, the interviewer has flexibility in being able to add, delete, or rework both topical ideas and questions, allowing the interviewer to explore "the living stage." Berg simplified some of the complexities of conducting interviews into ten commandments.

> Never begin an interview cold; remember your purpose; present a natural front; demonstrate aware hearing; think about appearance [as is consistent with the cultural context of vision discussed in Chapter One]; interview in a comfortable place; don't be satisfied with monosyllabic answers; be respectful; practice, practice, and practice some more; and be cordial and appreciative. (pp. 57-58)

Interviewing blind informants on videotape introduced a new challenge to the research process. When videotaping—if the tapes are to be used beyond documentation for research dissemination—the interviewer avoids conversation encouragers such as verbal cues of "uh huh," "I see" and "yes" and touch such as a hand placed on the informant's shoulder. Words, sounds, or body parts jutting in from off-camera distract viewers and interrupt the willing suspension of disbelief, reminding them that the tale is the product of a research interview with a person who is not included in the capture frame. With sighted informants, the interviewer relies on nonverbal cues to encourage conversation. The interviewer nods, smiles, shrugs, and raises one's eyebrows. Of course, the blind interlocuter does not see these cues.

I resorted to explaining my absence of verbal presence in the conversation between my comments and questions; before each first interview with an informant, I explained that I would be silent while he or she was speaking, but assured that I would indeed be listening. While comfort with silence is a learned skill of interviewers, in that many new researchers unintentionally truncate informant input by jumping in with their own comment or question, interviewing blind learners pushed interview technique even further with positive consequences. There were numerous instances in which I assumed that a *monologue* was concluded, paused to allow silence to confirm my interpretation and then opened my mouth to interject (which of course would have cued a sighted interlocuter to end his or her turn)—and the interviewee continued, often with key insights. I further reflected on how even seemingly neutral verbal encouragers such as "uh huh" are often interpreted as agreement rather than request for conversation continuance, and thus the interviewer unintentionally promotes yea-saying. Interviewing blind learners on camera necessitated intensified comfort with silence that promoted interlocuter contribution.

Qualitative researchers have been careful to distinguish the type of interview informing their research, and thus to ensure consistency with one's research philosophy, ontology, and epistemology. Neuman (1997) differentiated between survey and field interviews, describing the latter as more flexible, individualized, open-ended, jointly controlled, and contextual. Field interviews, deriving from ethnographic approaches, are often further defined as interactive. The essence of interactive interviews are that they: (a) are grounded on trust between the interviewer and research participant (Ellis, Kiesinger, & Tillman-Healy, 1997); (b) promote sharing of perceptions and experiences by both the interviewer and the participant (Neuman); (c) are not single events, but instead engage the interlocuters in multiple conversations that build on one another and unfold over time (Ellis, Kiesinger, & Tillman-Healy; Neuman) and; (d) involve a sharing of the interview transcripts between the interviewer and the participant. The interviewer "interrupts" the transcripts with questions, comments, and possible interpretations, and then transmits these back to the participant initiating an iterative exchange and interpretive process.

Within this research, initial interviews lasted between 1½ to 2½ hours in duration. They were loosely structured by the following themes: (a) demographics of the experience (year, institution, program, learning objectives, type of learning moderation system, number of students); (b) what it was like to be a blind online learner; (c) identification and affiliation with organized blind and professional organizations; (d) philosophical and social orientation to blindness; (e) comprehension of concepts presented through imagery such as metaphors; (f) strengths of the learning experience; (g) interaction and sense of community with classmates and instructor; (h) barriers and challenges to online learning; (i) impact of blindness on the learning experience; (j) relative accessibility of course content and communication tools; (k) adaptations to the course content and/or delivery; (l) assistive devices used by the student; (m) perceived impact of online learning on the inclusion or segregation of blind learners; and (n) impact of the learning experience on the accomplishment of educational objectives, career preparation, and transferable skills.

Rationale for Videography

The interviews were simultaneously conducted and videotaped by the researcher. A videographer was not used for two reasons. First, a one-on-one conversation protected the intimacy dynamic and the camera often was forgotten as the exchange progressed. Second, the realities of a limited budget were that professional videography was not an option. Instead, the researcher set the video camera up on a tripod.

The interviews were videotaped for four reasons. First, planned redundancy of communication modes facilitates accessible information. Burgstahler (2002) defined universal design as "the design of products and environments to be usable by all people, to the greatest extent possible, without the need for adaptation or specialized design" (p. 1). Negroponte (1995) explained that producing information in bits (e.g., digital video) rather than atoms (transcribed tapes) allows the user to pull the information in the desired format, rather than the producer pushing it in a medium that may not be functional. Within their 16 tips for online learning, Coombs and Banks (2000) advised designers to build-in multiple communication modes (planned redundancy). Capturing the interviews in a digital format facilitated production such that the research information may be accessed via speech, image with closed captioning, text-only and a combination, thus making it accessible to all users including those who are blind or deaf.

Second, infusing the technology into the research context facilitated a research product that was more likely to interest, intrigue, and engage. Gladstone (personal communication, March 7, 2003) commented that researchers are beginning to study the low frequency with which academic publications are actually read. With the publication expectations of academics and the World Wide Web further contributing to the overwhelming proliferation of print resources, video presentation might position this research product as unique, and thus increase the chances that the knowledge will be shared.

Third, video technologies provide a means of demonstration. Mayer (2001) wrote that learners demonstrate better retention and transfer when lessons are presented in words and pictures. Within this research, one of the interview probes concerned adaptive technologies. As a result, each of the research participants demonstrated one or more adaptive technologies. While their description was informative, actually hearing the speed of the synthesized voice of the screen reader, and watching the interface move off of the screen when using a screen enlarger has the potential to be more educative for an audience with vision and hearing.

Fourth, videotaping the interviews allowed participants to express their thoughts in their own voices. Flat paper transcripts, even interpreted into a coherent narrative, cannot capture the disdain, irony, humour, and cadence of the research informants. Whereas a sighted person primarily uses personal appearance to receive a sense of the person, the research participants shared that they primarily use the voice. Because they are practiced in voice discernment, the blind viewers were particularly pleased to hear the actual research participants expressing themselves.

Follow-up Correspondence

Subsequent to each face-to-face interview, a minimum of three e-mail correspondences occurred with each of the seven participants. Both the researcher and the participants initiated correspondence. The researcher initiated correspondence with each of the seven participants in three instances. First, detailed reading of the transcripts in relation to each of the seven initial conversations revealed gaps, dialectical interpretations, and potential thematic relationships that required further elaboration. Second, questions emerged from the literature and LISTSERV participation. Third, drafts of all conference papers, dissertation chapters, and video scripts were sent to each of the participants asking for feedback, input and discussion prior to finalizing.

Coding, Analysis, and Interpretation

Using iMovie, the videoclips of the interviews were interwoven and edited to construct four videos presenting: (a) each of the seven participants in turn introducing themselves and briefly describing what it is like to be a blind online learner; (b) issues of online learning in a disability studies context, such as debate as to whether online learning is a form of inclusion or segregation; (c) an interview with the experts on online learning, Norman Coombs and Dick Banks, of Equal Access to Software and Information; and (d) sixteen tips for the design and instruction of interactive online learning. To the extent possible with personal computer editing software, particular attention was directed to the audio presentation including sound levels, distinction between voices (e.g., alternating between male and female) and background musical and sound effects. The videotapes were produced on DVD. DVD production allowed information to be accessed in audio-only, video-only (with subtitles), and audiovisual format to accommodate the needs of people with sensory impairments.

The interviews were transcribed so that interpretation could be facilitated through the manipulation of videoclips and printed text. The interview transcripts were coded using Emerson, Fretz, and Shaw's (1995) methods of open coding, memoing and reflections. First, each text transcript was read-through multiple times line-by-line. Notes were made along the margins identifying content areas and potential themes. Memos were then added in a different color pen. Memos identified reflections, questions to pursue, associations with the literature and comparisons and contrasts between respondents. Second, the transcripts were reprinted. Each was printed on a unique color of paper. The transcripts were then manually cut and pasted together again according to themes across the transcripts. The patched transcripts were again read-through line-by-line, once again writing codes, memos, and reflections in the margins.

Upon completion of transcript coding, Alvesson and Sköldberg's (2000) quadri-reflexive framework grounded the research analysis. This particular approach to reflexive methodology integrates four types of reflection: (a) interaction with empirical material, (b) interpretation, (c) critical interpretation, and (d) discourse analysis. Alvesson and Sköldberg described their particular research approach as being conducted "from an emancipatory cognitive interest which critically interprets various empirical phenomena, with the purpose of stimulating self-reflection and overcoming the blockages of established institutions and modes of thought" (p. 128).

In keeping with this model, the empirical material was gathered through interviews and follow-up correspondence with blind online learners. In chapter 5, each of the informants' stories is presented individually. Chapter 6 presents an interpretation of these stories in accordance with the three research questions. What it is like to be a blind online learner is addressed through a series of grids. For example, overall evaluative perception of the online learning experience formed one axis of the grid, with the students' prior computer experience and the use of adaptive technologies on the other axes. The response to the second question regarding best design characteristics of online learning was informed through analyzing the transcripts to determine which of Coombs and Banks (2000) 16 tips for online learning resonated with the informants' descriptions of their experiences. The third question regarding the impact of online learning was addressed through checking themes emerging within the literature with the informants and by direct unprompted themes emerging within the interviews. Chapter 7 presents a reexamination of the interview transcripts through a critical theoretical perspective. Critical interpretation required reflection regarding who was included and excluded as informants, and explored themes of affiliation with blindness agencies and/or the organized blind (e.g., National Federation of the Blind) in Canada and the United States, and a social philosophical perspective on the desirability of online learning as informed by Postman's (2003) critical questions. In chapter 8, reflection on text production and language use was guided through application of social constructionist accounts of the matrix of blindness. Particular methods to ensure that the language of the research paid due attention to both the reflection and construction of meaning included: (a) sharing the interpretation of the interviews with the participants through reciprocal text interruption and an iterative/building model of interpretation, and (b) through conducting the interviews in an interactive manner. The responses to two open-ended questions were interpreted. Participants were asked to share whatever they would like about themselves and participants were asked what it is like to be a blind online learner. Analysis pursued, for example, at what point discussion of blindness emerged within their responses.

Summary

In summary, research into blind online learners was conducted through qualitative inquiry in the interpretive domain. Three questions guided the inquiry: (a) what is it like to be a blind student enrolled in online learning; (b) what design characteristics best facilitate learning for blind students; and (c) what is the impact of blind students engaged in online learning. Seven blind online learners were recruited and interviewed. The initial interviews were interactive face-to-face conversations. The initial interviews were videotaped. Follow-up correspondence was conducted through e-mail. Both the videoclips and paper transcripts of the conversations were manipulated. Transcripts were coded and memos added. Analysis was grounded in Alvesson and and Sköldberg's (2000) quadri-reflexive framework. Consistent with this model, four types of reflection informed the analysis: (a) interaction with empirical material, (b) interpretation, (c) critical interpretation, and (d) discourse analysis.

CHAPTER 5

THE STORIES

Seven Online Learners (Who are Blind)

INTRODUCTION

Analysis of this research is grounded by Alvesson and Sköldberg's (2000) quadri-reflexive framework. The first stage in the analysis is interaction with the empirical material. The empirical material, in this case, consisted of print transcripts and videoclips of face-to-face interactive interviews and print-outs of online correspondence with seven adults who are blind, use adaptive technologies to access computer information and interaction, and have enrolled in (not necessarily completed) a minimum of one online course.

This chapter presents each online learner in turn. The informants were given the opportunity to validate the stories. The intention of this chapter is to inform what it is like to be a blind online learner through the sometimes diverse and other times common experiences and perspectives of seven adults. As well as constructing new knowledge in the unresearched overlap between blindness and online learning from the perspective of the learner, the two categories (blind and online learner) were also considered discretely. Goals in this regard were to story the lived experience

Seeing Beyond Blindness, 61–96

of being blind and the experience of being an online learner. The characteristic of blindness sometimes impacted the informants' responses to what it is like to be an online learner, but the interview content much more often had nothing to do with blindness and everything to do with learning and the role of student.

Each online learner is biographically presented. In the course of the interviews, each learner was asked to share whatever he or she wanted about his or her life story. Some participants chose to reveal more personal information than others. Within the personal story, each participant's experience with computers was further queried. Interviewees were asked when they started using computers and why, and how proficient they now see themselves. The analysis then focused on the experience of online learning. The demographics of the online experience and evaluative perceptions of that experience are presented.

To avoid duplication of information, redundant details that are provided in relation to earlier presented interviewees are not subsequently repeated. For example, adaptive technologies and the process of preparing an assignment using such technologies are described in detail in the first section presenting Madeline's story and experiences. Five of the six other respondents use many of the same technologies such as screen-reading software. These technologies are not described in detail again within their stories and experiences. Additional technologies and discrepancies in the way in which they are used are presented throughout.

The seven online learners are presented in order of the nature and level of their online experience. The chapter opens with Madeline who completed a master's level degree through a blended model in which some of the courses were completed face-to-face through short concentrated-time study institutes and the majority of the courses were delivered online. Matthew is presented next. His degree is in process. He is completing courses toward a master's level degree through a blended model. Martin is in the process of completing an associate arts degree in which some of the courses are delivered online and others face-to-face. Sarah is a preprogram student. At the time of her interview, she was in the process of completing her third online course. She will apply these courses toward an entirely online master's degree program. Bernice completed an online course through Equal Access to Software and Information, a private university-based educational company. Through the same organization, Deborah completed an early offering of a noninteractive online course. Finally, Shannon enrolled in an online cooking course through private industry. Shannon successfully signed-up for the course and then withdrew. The intrigue and universality of Shannon's story comes in her vivid descriptions of being a new computer user.

Madeline

Madeline is a Canadian. She and her husband have two sons who are now university students. Madeline prides herself on active involvement in the grade-school experience of her sons. She progressed from a role on the local parent advisory committee to serving as the district parent advisory representative, and was then elected to the school board where she served three terms.

Madeline describes herself as being blind all of her life due to a condition called Retinopathy of Prematurity. Madeline was born almost 3 months premature. Madeline is 50 years old and was therefore treated within the confines of the medical knowledge of the 1950s. One of the theories is that too much oxygen was pumped into the incubators of premature babies.

Madeline began her education in a school for the blind, where she completed grades 1 through 10, and then went to her neighborhood high school for Grades 11 and 12. Madeline then went to university and earned a music degree, subsequently performing as a musician for 20 years. When Madeline decided to complete a master's degree program to become a teacher of the visually impaired, she had to first complete a bachelor's of education degree. She completed a 60-credit program earning a degree in secondary music from September 1999 to July 2000. That same July, she started the first two courses toward her master's degree. She earned her master's degree in 2002. Madeline's goal is to "establish early intervention systems … for children who are blind or visually impaired or who have additional disabilities."

Madeline has been using the computer for approximately 13 years. She started when her work for the school board required her to read and synthesize a great deal of print material. She can download items as directed. She describes herself as "pretty good" at navigating the World Wide Web and at word processing. She does not recall all of the key-stroke commands for upper level word processing layout features. She does not install software nor troubleshoot when the computer does not perform functions as expected. Madeline does not consider it "worth her time" to further develop her computer competency as she is married to a "senior systems analyst" who works within the human service industry.

Madeline uses adaptive technologies to access computer information and communication. She estimates that she has $25,000 worth of equipment in her home office. Some of the equipment is relatively inexpensive such as a scanner. N. Coombs and D. Banks (personal communication, March 19, 2003) observed that the price of software and equipment comes down as it is adopted beyond the disability community to mainstream use. Scanners are now widely used by people wanting to post materials such as photographs onto the World Wide Web, or who do not have access to digital copies of print materials in order to edit. Specialized scanning software that is compatible with a synthesized voice reader, on the other hand, is not used by the mainstream public and thereby costs approximately $1,100.

Madeline uses a hand-held Braille display called a Braille Lite that is priced at approximately $8,000. The Braille Lite has a Braille keyboard, a refreshable 40-character Braille display of raised pins, and an extensive memory so that entries can be read back through the display and/or recorded on paper through attachment to a Braille embosser. Madeline uses both a Braille embosser and a regular printer.

Madeline's computer has a monitor so that her husband or sons can also use it, and so that they can assist Madeline visually when she has questions about the display. Madeline does not use a mouse and thereby needs to know keystroke commands. Her keyboard is not adapted in any way. She accesses her computer through JAWS screen-reading software. The version Madeline uses costs approximately $1,100. When the computer is turned on, JAWS opens automatically, so that whatever the software can read of the display is spoken aloud through a synthesized voice. The gender, tone, and speed of the voice can be altered.

Madeline explained that "if you are blind or visually impaired and a non-print reader, then it's going to take you longer to do the work." She described her own personal experience as confirming this time factor that she has read about through her studies in education of the visually impaired. Madeline explained that it often takes a longer time to obtain the materials. Instructors are seldom prepared with alternate format texts in advance of the course. Whereas the sighted student can go to a bookstore or online and order the assigned text, the blind student either has to wait for the same text to be read onto tape, be released in a digital format, or transcribed into Braille, or scan the entire text herself. If accessing the text through self-scanning, she then has to correct numerous scanning errors. It then takes longer to read the text. People reading Braille can improve their words-per-minute rate through practice, and through learning advanced levels or grades of Braille that use increasing numbers of contractions, or shortened characters that stand for full words. However, as Braille does not allow skimming or many other speed-reading techniques, reading Braille is generally more time consuming than reading text. Reading is particularly slowed when accessing books on tape. Madeline explained that you can speed up the rate of the tape. "But the thing is that you cannot find a specific page and it just about drives you crazy."

Madeline explained that her student rate of assignment production is also slowed by the redundant task of preparing materials in both print and Braille.

> And it takes longer to print it and get it into accessible format for someone else to read. You're re-doing everything you're doing. Because everything I am doing, I am doing in Braille and then I have to get it into print.

Madeline described step-by-step, the preparation of an assignment. While listening to a book on tape, she takes digital format Braille notes using her handheld Braille Lite. She carefully labels the notes so that she can return to text on a given topic or chapter. She then makes a paper copy of her notes by hooking her Braille Lite to her Braille embosser. She reads over the Braille notes several times and then uses her Braille Lite to record her thoughts, ideas and experience relative to the text. She makes a paper copy of these notes using her embosser. She then drafts her assignment on her Braille Lite so that she can read the refreshable Braille display while in the process of writing. She once again makes a paper copy. Braille format texts are many more pages than their equivalent print editions, and the Braille paper is larger and thicker. Madeline said, "downstairs on my shelves, I have binders and binders and binders of all of the notes that I've taken from all of the books that I've read from all of my courses." She uses the paper copies of the text notes, her reflective notes, and her draft paper to inform the next draft which she keys into the computer. She listens to the draft using the JAWS screen-reading software, and corrects heard errors. She then makes a paper copy using the embosser to read a full-paper copy of the draft. She finds and corrects errors, and makes insertions, deletions, and reorganization of sections on the computer. She listens again for formatting. She then makes a print version for face-to-face assignment submission, or e-mails an electronic version for online course assignments.

In 2002 Madeline graduated from the University of British Columbia with a master's in special education with a concentration in blindness and visual impairment qualifying her to be a teacher of the visually impaired from birth through to Grade 12. There were eight students in Madeline's cohort. Most were from British Columbia, with one from Ontario. Madeline was the only student with an identified disability. The program was delivered using a blended model. The program was 2 years in duration, with online courses offered from September through June, on-campus courses for the summer semester, and concentrated-time study institutes in the spring for completion of joint projects. Seven of the courses were delivered online.

Madeline answered the question—"What is it like to be a blind online learner?" with an evaluation of her experience. She replied that it was more positive than negative.

> There were aspects of it I really liked and aspects of it I didn't like. I had the advantage of doing part of my program online and part on-campus. And the things I really liked about it was that I could work on it on my own time. I could work at my own pace. And if it was really horrible out, and awful and raining, I didn't have to travel. I found that really reduced the stress. The thing that I didn't like (and this surprised me), I thought that I would never say that I had a problem with self-discipline ever, with getting the work done. I had a bit of a problem, and a minor problem really with motivating myself to do it. That might happen maybe once or twice a month. But I thought that being around other people doing the same thing and being in the class, and having to psych yourself up to be in there communicating with people and talking with other people while you're doing your work. That part of it I missed a little bit. That surprised me. But generally, I would say that there were more advantages than disadvantages. The other thing that I found good from the perspective of being blind was that I had most things on my computer, well at least *most* things on my computer. That was a lot better than going to class and dealing with worksheets that the teacher decided to do up at the last minute. So it was accessible if it can be set-up right.

In summary, the positive elements of online learning from Madeline's perspective were the accessibility of the course content, the anytime/anyplace convenience including the comfort of working from home rather than enduring weather elements, and the self-pacing of the learning. The negative elements were the absence of a designated learning time and place with the physical presence of a community of learners germane to the educational experience. These absences occasionally resulted in a motivational challenge.

Madeline explained that her cohort was a pilot group. Prior to this particular offering of the program, the entire program was delivered face-to-face. Madeline explained that the blended model was developed to "accommodate the fact that most people were working full-time or part-time and also that people were from other parts of the country." Madeline is an advocate of the blended model. She believes that program designers are "asking for trouble" if they design purely online programs. She described the advantages of the blended model.

> I think we had the best of both. I don't think we could have interacted online well, if we didn't know each other personally. The course started in the summer with the Foundations course and the Braille course, so we did all get to know each other personally and could establish some relation-

> ships. I don't think we would have had the discussions, the in-depth discussions, the problem-solving, the sharing if one of us hit a crisis. I don't think we could have done that if we hadn't known each other personally. And if we would have just had it in-class, then we wouldn't have had the participants because people wouldn't have been able to leave their full-time jobs and done the program. So it was definitely, definitely the best way.

In summary, the main benefit of the face-to-face component of the blended model, from Madeline's perspective, is the personal interaction creating a foundation for online discussion and sustained relationships promoting collegial support. The benefit of the online component is the anytime, anyplace convenience allowing for adequate program enrolment.

The online courses were offered using Web sites and e-mail correspondence. They were not designed or delivered through learning moderation systems or other packaged courseware. Madeline provided a step-by-step description of an online course. First, the instructor would send an e-mail to each of the learners through a LISTSERV stating that a new lesson was posted, and providing a URL and an assignment due-date. The link would have a banner with the number and title of the lesson and resource information. The information was delivered via original text, scanned-in readings, links to other Web sites, directions to read designated chapters from a previously mailed-out text, or a combination thereof. Each lesson Web site also included an assignment. Madeline described the process of using one such online lesson.

> So you'd do your readings, and then you'd consider your assignment in terms of what you've read. And the assignment would ask you to consider a certain situation in terms of what you've read. And usually what [the instructor] would do, is she'd give you a scenario such as a student is having areas of difficulty, and ask what you would do as a teacher to try to accommodate that. So you would talk about how you would use what you had read, and your own ideas, and how you would put it into practice and for instance, a person's having trouble learning how to dress appropriately and comb their hair for school. So you'd read the book. And maybe the book would say that you need to build in some home time with that student to help the student organize their things and maybe you need to show the parents how to help that student to dress appropriately. And maybe you need to show the parents that the child needs to learn how to dress himself. So everything looks appropriate. And you take all of those things that you're reading about, and take into account your own ideas, and build that into your assignment.

Using the process as described above, Madeline completed her assignments and then e-mailed them to her instructor. In turn, the instructor conveyed grades and comments via e-mail.

E-mail was the primary communication tool used throughout the online courses. Madeline described e-mail as providing a sense of connectedness amongst the students and instructor.

> Generally, we communicated through e-mail. And we always knew that if something private needed to be discussed that we could send a private e-mail rather than through the LISTSERV. But I don't ever recall, to my knowledge that never happened. It was a really close group.

At one point in the program, the instructor attempted to use a bulletin board for interaction. The experiment was unsuccessful. The students could not navigate the bulletin board. Madeline described the deleterious effect.

> I think the only time I ever remember feeling isolated was when we tried to use technology that wasn't working, like the bulletin board. I felt out of the loop because I thought that I was the only one who couldn't make it work. And I felt that it was my fault because I didn't have enough knowledge, or I wasn't doing it right, or it was an accessibility issue. It was frustrating when I was trying to do my work.

Inability to navigate the bulletin board was not a result of Madeline being blind. She was the only blind learner, and yet the troubles with the communication tool were unanimous.

> I found out, when we started talking about it that it wasn't just me. The others were having the same experience. So that's why we decided to go back to the old LISTSERV. Even though the bulletin board would have provided an archive that other people could have used, that would have provided information that would have been very valuable, it wasn't working for *us*. And if it wasn't working for us, then we said, "No, we'll go back to our old original LISTSERV." And that, to me, resulted in us not feeling isolated.

When asked whether she would recommend communication tools other than e-mail within course design, Madeline replied that e-mail functioned effectively and fulfilled the interactive function. If additional communication tools were warranted within the course design, then they would need to be tested for compatibility with adaptive technologies such as screen reading software, and each student would require access to individual training in use of the tools.

In summary, Madeline is a middle-aged woman who recently completed an online master's degree in special education through a blended model. Madeline is blind and primarily uses JAWS screen reading software for accessibility. She evaluated the online component as more positive than negative. The online courses were delivered through discrete lessons, each with its own Web site. E-mail coordinated through a LISTSERV was the communication tool of choice.

Matthew

Matthew is a Canadian. He described himself as introspective, enjoying observing the world and reflecting upon it as a "true introvert." He is a step-grandparent through a former relationship, and maintains a close relationship with his stepson and stepdaughter. He enjoys alternative films.

Matthew is the personal empowerment coordinator for an Independent Living Resource Centre. He described their mandate as "encourag[ing] people with disabilities to make their own individual choice of living independently, and how they'd like to live independently." The program is consumer driven, meaning that many of their staff and board members have some form of disability. He described his role as "advisor in terms of human rights, and ... bridging a person from becoming entirely powerless to empowering themselves." Former careers include developing barrier-free access to national parks and national historic sites and working for the Canadian National Institute for the Blind.

Matthew is legally blind and has low vision. He has an eye condition called Retinitis Pigmentosa that he described as "extremely limited fields." He explained,

> It's inherited. I can trace it back three generations. And the first symptom is you lose a lot of night vision, because it affects the rods of the retina and it slowly deteriorates towards the central part of the retina. And I'm at the point now where it's starting to affect my cones, my color vision, my detail vision a lot, because it has deteriorated to the point where it's just a pinpoint of vision. But consequently it's affected my contrast, my contrasting vision.

Matthew's mother has the same condition and was watchful of her son's vision. The first behavioral indication of low vision occurred when Matthew was 5 years old and began to "hang back" in movie theaters. Several times throughout the conversation, Matthew reiterated that his visual impairment is "just part of my being." He used a metaphor to elaborate.

> I heard a beautiful analogy one time from a gentleman who has a doctorate and he has the same eye condition.... A person with a disability is like a rock sitting on a piece of glass. And if you can hold up that glass and look through it and see all of the different perspectives from the reflection off the rock, that's like seeing a person with a disability, because that disability is just part of your being. If you don't accept that, if you feel that that disability

> is constantly in the way, all you're doing is picking up that rock and hitting that glass.

Matthew described his visual impairment as giving him an appreciation for diversity.

His vision began to have a recognizable impact when Matthew was in grade school. Matthew went to his neighborhood school through Grade 4. He was then transferred to what was then called a "sight saving class" which tongue-in-cheek, Matthew described as not saving any of his sight. He appreciated the opportunity to meet peers who were experiencing similar obstacles to "compare notes and say, 'well, how do you deal with this problem? This is the way I do it." He completed Grades 5 to 9 through this class, and was then "reintegrated" into the high school designated for his neighborhood. Through attending terms at both the local university and local college, and taking transfer credits through a distance education campus, Matthew graduated with a bachelor of general studies with social science content in fields such as geography.

Matthew described numerous instances of inaccessibility throughout his schooling. He described the frustration of not being able to see the blackboard when the teachers demonstrated mathematical concepts. He relayed one particular instance of inaccessibility in post-secondary.

> And it was a course on meteorology.... I remember taking that course and struggling with it. I was doing okay. I was getting a "C" through the course. But one of the tutorials, the tutorials regularly, was to go out to the weather station there, read the instruments, record your readings, and of course, analyze those readings. Well, I couldn't read the instruments. And I went in to my Prof and I said, "I can't handle this. Is there some way that I can learn the theory and pass in terms of learning the theory, but not actually physically going out and reading the instruments?" He said, "Well [Matthew] if you had a 'B' or better, I might consider that. But I'm not going to let you do that." Now today, he wouldn't be allowed to do that. He wouldn't have been allowed to not give me that accommodation. So I ended up, at that time it was too late in the session to withdraw from the course. I ended up just sacrificing that course. I ended up with an "F" in the course, which was my only "F" toward my degree.

Matthew cited accessibility as one of the advantages of computer mediated education. The user can more easily manipulate digital information and through use of adaptive technologies, the accessibility of digital information is enhanced.

At this point, Matthew navigates the computer through a monitor and mouse, although he expects that his declining vision will require use of screen reading software and keyboard commands in the future. He moves a handheld magnifier over the monitor and keyboard to enlarge the image. He also has ZoomText screen enlarging software installed on his computer. He described that "you can only perceive about a quarter of the screen at the magnification that I use on it at one time so I'm constantly scanning with the mouse." He further described,

> If I can play with the size of the image, I'll reduce it, which is really ironic. You'd think you'd want to enlarge it, but I want to reduce it so that I get the full image within that magnified section of the screen. That's always difficult as well. But I should be thankful, because I probably couldn't use the computer at all if ZoomText wasn't there.

Matthew recognizes ZoomText as an essential adaptive technology enabling him to use the computer, but is sometimes frustrated by navigating spreads of information of which he can only see a portion at a time.

Matthew began using the computer in 1990. He described himself as an "anachronism" saying that prior to that "I barely even touched a computer." He judges himself "very proficient" in applications such as Microsoft Word and in using word processing generally. He would like to learn Microsoft PowerPoint, and stated, "I'm absolutely terrible in using something like Excel or in using tables, even compiling a table or doing graphs and graphics." Matthew explained that he self-assessed his limited computer proficiency as a factor when considering online learning. When asked whether he would choose online or traditional education if his program was offered via both models, he replied,

> I probably would have chosen online simply because of the time constraints I have with my work. However, if I was not working, interestingly, I probably would have chosen face-to-face, simply because I'm not confident in the use of the computer. I'm such an anachronism. I'm still back there almost in the quill stage—not that far, but I'm still learning a lot about the computer. I'm not totally confident in my skills.

Matthew is currently enrolled in the master of continuing education program through the University of Calgary. He is specializing in leadership and development. He began the program in June 2002. There are 23 students in Matthew's cohort. At the time of our conversation, Matthew was in the process of completing his fourth course, which is his second online. Because Matthew is employed full-time, and because reading with a hand-held magnifier decreases his reading rate, he enrolls in one course per term.

The program is designed on a blended model. There is a 3 week spring or summer institute each year. Students taking a full course load will participate in two such institutes, one at the beginning of their program and the other between the 2 program years. Two courses are delivered through each institute. The other courses are delivered online. Matthew discussed the various pros and cons of the face-to-face and online components.

> I'm a true introvert. When I'm sitting in a classroom, until I really get to know people, I'm not that expressive. I don't offer a lot of ideas. It probably took me a good half-week to a week when I was taking my institute to feel comfortable enough to express my true points. But ironically, when I'm at home, I feel really quite isolated. I can't say that I don't enjoy the online learning part of it. I really do. I just love the ability to really think out my message before I post it and actually re-read it and spell check. Thank heaven for spell-check; it's one technology I love because my spelling used to be terrible. So, in some ways, in terms of the literature and being able to conceptualize my thoughts before my big mouth is beneficial at home. But I truly enjoy those three-week face-to-face classes. And I'm so looking forward to next June when we can get together again. And I think a lot of my colleagues would feel that way as well.

The adjective that Matthew used with the most frequency to describe his online program of studies is "fascinating." This adjective is applied to the interaction between what he perceives to be the intriguing and introspection-provoking content, and the means of delivery. From Matthew's perspective, the advantages of the online component are the increased time delay between question and response thereby promoting reflection and facilitating review of the literature, and the capacity for editing and spell-checking. The advantage of the face-to-face component is the collegiality and enjoyment of being together. The disadvantage of the online component is the feeling of isolation provoked by studying alone. The disadvantage of the face-to-face component is the introverted student's feeling of trepidation and thus infrequency and delay in offering input.

Matthew's courses were designed and delivered using First Class courseware. The lessons and other course components are all grouped together and accessed through one URL. Matthew described the course structure and his interaction with the site.

> I do check First Class everyday.... It's a series of icons that you see in the course. Each icon will lead you into a different folder. And for example, the course that I'm taking now, there's one folder—"introductory"—an introduction to the course itself. That's where you put your general postings as to any questions that you have about the course itself. This course has four modules in it, so there will be four icons below that—modules one, two, three and four. And during the first three weeks of the program (module one is three weeks), you go into module one and you put your postings in there. So you click on module one and it opens up and it gives you a listing of all of the conversations that have taken place and all of the postings up to

> that point. And we term them as red flags. It is truly a little red flag. If there is a red flag showing up you click on that and you open it and that will give you the message. And sometimes I'll go home in the evening and click on that module one and there will be about a hundred red flags that I will have to go through. So I'm clicking away and reading, and clicking away and reading. Probably three hours.

The majority of course readings are off-line. Students purchase texts or books of readings in advance of the course either through the local university bookstore or through ordering by mail. The students submit their assignments electronically through an assignment drop-box or sometimes as e-mail attachments.

Interaction is facilitated through the communication tools of e-mail, bulletin boards, and synchronous text-based chat. Matthew was referring to the asynchronous bulletin board when describing the red flags. The instructor creates a number of topic streams. The student selects a topic stream and then posts a message either as a discrete entry or as a reply to one of the other postings. If posted as a reply, the message is indented from the source posting. The postings can be arranged on the screen via a toggle button to either display according to topic (threaded) or by date of posting. In bulletin boards administered through First Class software, a red flag next to the posting indicates that the user has not yet read the message. The red flag does not appear after the message has been clicked-on once. Matthew experienced the bulletin board as accessible.

Synchronous text-based chat requires the instructor and/or students to designate what date and time they will meet in a virtual chat-room. The students key-in text into a box on the lower portion of their display. This box can only be seen by the single user. The text appears in the upper shared portion of the screen on all of the monitors of the participants logged into the chat-room, in the order in which the users click-on "enter." Matthew did not experience the synchronous chat as functional.

> With First Class, we can have synchronous communication where we have a chat. I find it really, really difficult because of course with my eye condition, I'm only picking up three or four words at a time. If you get eight people on a chat, they're clicking away, and they're giving message after message after message. And it scrolls up every time you get a new message on. So I'm concentrating on a line down here, and I get half-way through and the line scrolls up. And I have to go up and refocus on it, read it again, and of course it scrolls up again, because the third or fourth person comes in. So in terms of just having synchronous communication with text, it's very very difficult for me.

Matthew did not comment whether any of the other students in his cohort experienced the same frustrations with synchronous chat. The literature indicates that frustrations with the chat communication tool are not unique to learners with visual impairments. McNamee and Roberts (2002) reviewed 12 case studies of postsecondary online learning. These case studies were largely drawn from mainstream graduate education programs. They cited frequent mention of student frustration with adopting the technological functions of synchronous chat without training. They also cited a study suggesting, "when there are more than five people in one chat space, cognitive overload can occur stifling the problem solving process" (p. 4).

In summary of Matthew's story, Matthew is a middle-aged man enrolled in a program of studies leading to a master's degree in continuing education. The program is offered through a blended model, and at the time of the interview Matthew was enrolled in his second online course offered through First Class courseware. Matthew is visually impaired and primarily uses ZoomText software for accessibility. Matthew described the program of studies as "fascinating." He appreciates the convenience of the online component as he is employed full-time.

Martin

Martin is American. He is married and between him and his wife, they have nine grown children. He enjoys reading and attending conferences. He spent 15 years in cafeteria management in the state capital area, bringing him into contact with numerous legislators and other political figures.

Martin has been employed with the Iowa Department for the Blind since 1996. He works for a project titled "Accessible Step-by-Step Instruction Using Speech Technology" (ASSIST) whose mandate is to "teach blind people how to use computers and principally the Windows environment, and then popular Windows applications."

Martin has Retinopathy of Prematurity. He was born 6 weeks premature. Martin became affiliated with the National Federation of the Blind in the 1960s and has remained an active member. He explained,

> And one of the reasons is because I like the philosophy of blindness that the National Federation of the Blind espouses, which is basically that blindness really isn't a catastrophe—it's more a nuisance than anything else. It's just a part of you—it's a characteristic, I guess. It's who I am. I guess I like that philosophy that a blind person with proper training and opportunity can do the average job in the average place of business. As well as their sighted neighbour or better sometimes.

Martin's belief in the capacity of blind people given training and opportunity motivated him to develop his computer proficiency and then promote this proficiency in others.

Martin started learning to use computers in 1990 to catalyze a career change from food service management to finance and insurance. Martin self-taught himself to use DOS, then screen reading software, and then Windows and their applications. Since being hired to the Iowa Department for the Blind, Martin has contributed to the development of tutorials for numerous types and versions of screen reading software, Windows operating systems, and software such as Microsoft Word, Excel, and Access, as well as Internet Explorer and Microsoft Outlook. He is excited about the potential for the latest project that uses online learning to train blind individuals who would like to become Microsoft Office specialists.

Martin is enrolled in an associate arts degree program at the IAB College of Business. He started his first course toward an information technology degree 2 years ago. He started by taking two courses a quarter, and reduced his load to one per quarter finding it more feasible while employed full-time. To date, Martin has completed 15 courses, three of which were online. The college has a large number of "continuing education'" students who are studying while employed full-time. For that reason, they are in the process of developing increasing numbers of online courses to compliment face-to-face delivery. In the future, Martin believes that learners will be able to choose whether to take most of their courses face-to-face or online.

When asked what it is like to be a blind online learner, Martin answered by evaluating the experience.

> I think the best answer to that question is just to say that it has really liberated me as a student. I'm a part-time student because I work full-time at the Iowa Department for the Blind. And so, I have a limited time that I can go physically to class. And I've done it, but when online classes became available at my school, then I tried those and it gave me real freedom. I was able to access the same information that the rest of the students accessed, do the assignments, submit them and so forth. So it really gave me a huge bunch of freedom. And I really enjoyed—so I didn't have to worry about having to take a night or two of my time and spend three-and-a-half to three hours and forty-five minutes in class.

Martin evaluated his own experience of online learning positively. His words depict online learning as liberating, freeing, and accessible. Within this line of thinking his reference to access refers to life situation and roles and not to sensory limitations. He believes that the profile characteristics of a good candidate for online learning are employed full-time and a capacity for self-motivation, self-direction, and self-discipline.

Martin does not believe that online learning is the best option for all students. He believes that 20-something students benefit from the experience of the on-campus social interaction. Adding the factor of blindness, he believes that the social experience is particularly important, as it is more frequently avoided.

> We have clients at the Department, if they could avoid face-to-face contact with people, they'd do it. And, they would avoid all they could, getting out in the community, and having to travel to places they didn't know. Because they're not confident in themselves. So that is why we don't encourage online (basically online classes), because we don't want people to fall into that trap, and decide they're going to stay home and take their classes that way.

Pushing the conversation further, Martin was asked whether he believes that face-to-face is a better educational system than online for everyone. He responded positively, yet qualifying that it is simply not realistic for mature students who are employed full-time and have commitments such as family. The convenience of the online delivery outweighs the pedagogic and social advantages of face-to-face when a student fits the busy profile.

> I think really that face-to-face is really a better system for everybody. And the reason I say that is because—is because the interaction you achieve face-to-face. You know, I could sit in the classroom, and the instructor is talking about something, and somebody might make a point and say, "Oh, I want to respond to that." And with an online class, a lot of times, unless they're using an online chat, or something like that, you don't know for sure, the instructor doesn't do that much lecturing at all, as it were, so, it (online class) doesn't allow, I think, for as much interaction as a face-to-face class does. That's for anybody.

Martin believes that the interaction is reduced in an online course as compared to a face-to-face course. However, in his experience this does not translate to a feeling of isolation. When asked about his particular experience of interaction, he replied, "I've always enjoyed good interaction with students and teachers alike." He qualified that his own experience of positive interaction might be due to his computer proficiency. "And maybe it's just 'cause I'm so used to the Internet, 'cause I have used it for quite some time."

Martin lodges an additional criticism of online learning, in that his experience of online learning did not invite the expertise and interpretation of the course instructor to the extent of face-to-face delivery.

> Another thing with the online class is more than that, as you work on your assignments, you're more on your own than you are with the face-to-face, and what I mean by that, a lot of times, the instructor with your face-to-face class will go through the book, they'll lecture on the different chapters. You don't get that with an online class. Unless they choose to provide lecture notes, which a lot of times, at least mine have not. So, you miss a lot of that too. Because a lot of times, they'll throw up some little tidbits that the book doesn't have. Depending on your subject matter. So, there are advantages and disadvantages to this class. And it doesn't make any difference whether you're blind or sighted.

In summary, Martin's evaluation of online learning is intriguingly ambiguous. His life circumstances combined with the convenience of online learning make this option the most desirable. However, for people with more time, the social component, the opportunities for spontaneous interaction, and the interpretive editorial input of the instructor make face-to-face models a better educational practice.

The three online courses that Martin has taken to date have been offered through the Blackboard learning moderation system. Martin described what this courseware "looks like" and how he navigates the site using JAWS screen reading software.

> I go to what is called the Blackboard login screen, and what I've done is, I've created a short-cut to that on my desktop, so I can just get to that. And the screen comes up and I have to submit my user name and password and then press the log-in button. When the initial screen comes up then I have to choose a link to my particular course. And after I've done that, then I can choose either assignments or announcements or whatever I want to look at, that particular day. Or I can go to course documents and take a look at what's in there if I need to. So there are a lot of areas I can get to after I've gotten there. Once I read the announcements, if I need to do some participating in the discussion board, I just find that, press enter, in there, and create a new message if I need to, or respond to one, or whatever the case might be. And so, when I'm finished reading all of my messages that are on there, and downloading any files that I need to download, then I will just log-off and do whatever I can offline. And when it comes to submitting assignments, then I get back on the Blackboard platform and go to what's called the tools area and then digital drop-box and then I go to add-file and I could choose just, there's an add and a send file, and I could choose to add it to my drop-box area first, so I always know which files I have already done so I don't lose track of that. And after I've added the file, then I send it and the instructor gets that file. And there's always a record of the fact that the instructor got that file.

Interaction in Martin's courses was facilitated through three types of communication tools—bulletin boards, e-mail, and synchronous chat. Of the three, Martin prefers the bulletin board. He described enjoying the public nature of the bulletin board postings providing access to all students. He also enjoyed the flow of the threaded discussion. "Because then you can kind of follow a discussion through. If you start at the beginning, you can follow it through, read people's responses, and what have you."

Martin was unable to comment on the pedagogic (dis)advantages of synchronous chat, as he found this feature inaccessible. The version of speech reader he uses (JAWS for Windows 4.51) is incompatible with the version of Blackboard courseware used by his college (Blackboard version 5). He explained, "I can log into it. The instructor knows I've logged in, but that's all I can do. I can't read it." Martin was satisfied by the instructor's accommodation comprised of sending "basically the gist of what was said" through e-mail.

Summarizing Martin's story generally and with respect to online learning, Martin is a middle-aged man who is employed full time. His career work keeps his computer skills up-to-date. Martin is blind and primarily uses JAWS screen reading software to access the computer. He is in the process of completing an associate arts degree. To date he has taken three online courses offered via Blackboard courseware. He evaluates online learning positively given his life circumstances. The convenience of online learning is its best feature. For learners with more time, he believes that face-to-face models are better pedagogically and socially.

Sarah

Sarah lives in a Canadian town of 6,000 people. Education is valued within her family. Her husband has a master's degree. Her son recently graduated from medicine and will specialize in psychiatry. Her daughter has completed her master's degree and is now pursuing her doctorate in psychology.

Sarah has authored three books and is in the beginning stages of a fourth. One is a history text. The second book is comprised of insightful sayings about coping with stress. The third is informed by interviews with people who have experienced vision loss, and provides an interpretive approach to collective responses and diversity in perspective. The book in process will provide insight into what it is like to learn something new as an adult. Complimenting her experience as author, Sarah has led a support group, and is frequently asked to guest lecture. The interview with Sarah is grounded in her reflective disposition, her interpretations of learning experiences as she prepares for the authoring of her new book, and her interest in conversations as a means of informing inquiry.

Sarah was fully sighted until 17 years ago. She said, "I had hemorrhaging behind my eyes, just similar to macular degeneration, but not caused by that. And so the actual change happened immediately." The doctors tell her that her vision is now stable excepting the normal degeneration that happens with age. She described her current functional vision.

> In my right eye, I have motion vision, is what they tell me. And in my left eye, it is 20/400. That means that I can hold my hands out and I can't count how many fingers with either eye, if I hold my fingers out. And as I look at you, I can't really see your face. You're sitting what three or four feet away from me. So I don't have central vision at all.

Shortly after her vision loss, Sarah began using a closed-circuit television reader (CCTV) that might be envisioned as a personal overhead projector. An image or text is placed on the bottom plate and is projected onto the upper monitor. The user controls the contrast and the scale of enlargement. The CCTV allows Sarah to read two or three words on the screen at a time. In 2002 Sarah took a face-to-face course teaching her how to use JAWS screen reading software. She now prefers information in a digital format, as her reading rate is greatly accelerated using JAWS rather than using the CCTV. In addition, Sarah said that the CCTV reader "leaves me feeling rather sea-sick."

Sarah dedicated herself to a career as an elementary school teacher. She described her work as a calling and as a passion. She maintained her position as teacher for several years following her vision loss, and then decided to make a change. She maintained her classroom work without revealing her loss of vision to the children or parents—by using the CCTV, by inviting a supportive full-time volunteer into her classroom, and by what she labels "memory work," such as memorizing where the children sat and what they were wearing when they were up close so that she could identify them by the block of color when they were farther from her.

At the time of interview, Sarah was a preprogram student through Athabasca University. She was in the process of taking her third online course toward a program offered entirely online. Her plan is to complete several of the courses as a preprogram student and then transfer into the program. Taking the additional time factor of course completion resulting from her visual impairment into account, Sarah wants to enter the program with the prospect of completing it in a timely manner. She will graduate with a master's of arts in integrated studies. She will specialize in experiential learning with adults.

The three courses Sarah experienced at the time of the interview were conducted through mail-out packages and Web board courseware. When she transfers into the master's of arts in integrated studies program she will be using the Blackboard learning moderation system. Sarah described the course process. First, she registers for the course. Second, upon successful registration her e-mail address is forwarded to the course instructor who initiates online correspondence. The instructor e-mails with a message reading, "Here we are. We're on-board and this is where you find this, that and the other, and they give you a password to go into the program." Third, she receives a box via post that contains a printed course outline, textbooks, printed readings, and a schedule guide. Fourth, Sarah arranges for audiotaping of the print materials. If she receives the materials in time, Sarah takes them to the Canadian National Institute for the Blind, where a volunteer will complete the reading. If she does not receive the readings in sufficient advance of the course, one of her family members will read it for her.

Course interaction is conducted through bulletin board. From her perspective as teacher, Sarah commended the pedagogy of online interaction in terms of the promotion of critical thinking and problem solving.

> I prefer thinking about things in that online situation.... Let's say that there's a posting on the board that asks a question about something or other, I like the idea of being able to mull that over in my mind. And I will sometimes look at it, and I won't get back to it for half-a-day, before I actually form a response to it. I like to do things that way. To be able to sort of, 'this may be right, but that may be right, what do I really feel this, or do I really feel that? Oh, was there something I read or heard about that?' And I can go back and I can find that so that when I actually post a response, my response is probably a better response for having thought about it for that little while rather than having just been in the classroom, and saying, "Oh ya, I remember." And then rambling something off the top of my head. So to me, I feel that the online learning does give you more of an opportunity for critical thinking for sure. You know, to think critically through a situation rather than just pop-off with a little bit of knowledge and an instant response.

While Sarah cited the advantages of the asynchronous discussion, she experienced some of the courseware itself as inaccessible. She described the format and her means of accessing the postings.

> I haven't been able to negotiate the conference sites with my JAWS program. There's a posting, and then there are these different threads through the conference. Unless I go back to the beginning and I read them all. I haven't been able to figure out a way of getting the JAWS program to identify read from unread message. I haven't found a way to go through these threads. So every night, my husband and I sit down and go through the messages and he reads all these messages for me and he's able to see which

> is red and which is blue [distinguishing between read and unread postings] which is great.

When asked what her goal is in completing this degree, Sarah responded ambivalently and humorously. With laughter interspersed throughout her words, Sarah said,

> My plan—I'm not sure why I started. I'm not sure why I'm going to finish. I started because I do like to set new goals for myself. I found that really difficult with the onset of vision loss to find where my goals would be. I like to have a challenge and I think that this is a challenge. What would I do with it? I don't know. I would probably just put some letters after my name and say, "Here. I did this." No real practical purpose in doing this. I do like to learn. I'm enjoying the communication that this particular course has offered. I hope it will happen again in one of the other courses that I am doing.

Consistent with her life philosophy, her enrollment in the program began as a journey, or a quest of process, without a particular intentional outcome in mind. She explained,

> My daughter started searching around for a program that might be good for me, and she came across one on experiential learning and I was just so excited about that. All these adults who lose their sight at that particular point in life—really you're not prepared for anything. And the whole thing is learning by experience. I got in contact with … Athabasca University and found that I couldn't do that particular course. And by that time, I'd gone through about four months of trying to find out where I belonged with online learning, and couldn't do that course 'cause it was full. And I was so energized by the whole process that I thought, "Well, I just have to do something!" I registered in an adult learning course. It was just a really exciting experience! Using the screen reading program, because that was new, I worked at this practically every waking moment of the day.

The energy and excitement Sarah reported experiencing in anticipation of enrollment in online learning carried through her experience into her third online course. When asked if Athabasca University had an extension campus in her community, whereby she could take the same program face-to-face, which option she would choose, without hesitation Sarah replied "online."

> Because my community is six thousand people. I am out in my community pretty well every day. I'm out there saying, "Here I am. I am visually impaired." I don't need one more place that I'm going to do that. If I lived in the city, I would consider doing that as an extension course, where I was face-to-face with other people. I would consider that. I'm not sure. It would

depend on the other things that are involved with the course. A lot of instructors in a classroom, for instance, like to write on a board. If I'm in a face-to-face classroom, I don't see that. If they're choosing to write on a conference board on a computer, I can access that. In a classroom, sometimes the instructors will refer you to a textbook on a certain page. If I'm in a face-to-face classroom interaction, I can't open my textbook and find that page. Whereas if I'm at home, and the instructor says on the computer, look at such-and-such a page, I can take another half-an-hour to use means at my disposal to find that page, either by using my CCTV reader, or using a family member.

Sarah expressed considerable hesitation when she said that she might "consider" face-to-face courses. From her perspective, there are numerous advantages of online learning. First, digital information can be pulled in the format that best fits the needs of the learner. For example, Sarah can listen to the information using her screen reader. Classroom blackboard illustrations do not provide this option. Second, and related to the first, the asynchronicity of online learning provides time for the learner to use means to access the material. Third, she is able to maintain a level of anonymity. She described online presence as a form of "escapism." She discloses her visual impairment to the course instructor to avoid instances of inaccessibility. However, she avoids informing her student colleagues. She expressed that she appreciates the opportunity to engage in educational discussions without the stigma of visual impairment. She feels judged for her scholarship and not for what the public perceives as her (in)ability to cope as a visually impaired learner.

Sarah described an instance in which she felt forced to disclose her identity as visually impaired to her fellow learners. There are 25 students in her current course. She described them as a "particularly chatty group" as indicated by the number and length of the bulletin board postings. Tongue in cheek, she paraphrased multiple postings of one of the students. She said that he is "really enamoured with the technical aspect of working online and he was suggesting that we use HTML and do this and do that, and let's have some *fun* with this course." She described an increasing sense of confusion and frustration. One of the other learners posted a message reading, "Now if anyone has a problem with this, now's the time to speak up." Sarah described her posting in which she "spoke up" and her feelings regarding feeling forced to self-identify as disabled.

And I said, "Well, I just have to respond. Because this is *it*!" So I respond by saying that this was not in the original prerequisites for the course, and what are they all doing, and please stop because I'm legally blind and I can't see the screen anyway, and I'm just frustrated with this, and I'm speaking up! So, I went to bed and hardly slept that night at all having just burst out of

> my box in this way. Boom! Here I am! And had hoped to remain unidentified I guess, and thinking that this was one of the plusses of the course that I could stay, that I could be just another student with everybody else. So I was really upset by this whole thing of having to self-identify. It was really annoying to me. And frustrating and upsetting.

Forty-eight hours later a reply came personally to Sarah via e-mail. The student who had written the message about speaking up wrote an apology to Sarah. They began a scholarly acquaintance that expanded to include another woman. The triad was between Sarah, the second woman who lives several provinces away, and the third woman living in Italy. They jointly authored an assignment and made additional plans. The second woman became enamoured with accessible education and dedicated research to that topic. The acquaintance evolved to online friendship. Very few days go by that they do not correspond online. Time zones mean that the morning arrives earlier in Italy than in Canada. The woman living there starts her day by writing a chatty note to the other two via e-mail, and they begin their mornings by reading it. The three made plans to meet in person a few months following the interview with Sarah. In anticipation of this meeting, Sarah queried whether they would get along as well in person as they did online. She also commented that they knew different details about each other's lives than they would if they were friends outside the virtual realm. They did not know what each other looked like, and they did not know each other's socioeconomic status nor what kind of home each lived in. Yet, they knew each other's favorites, frustrations, and passions. Sarah e-mailed after their meeting to say that they got along famously and had made a date to get together again.

In summary, Sarah is a woman in her middle years living in a small Canadian community. Sarah has had low vision for the last 17 years, and uses a CCTV reader and JAWS screen-reading software to access text. At the time of the interview she was enrolled in her third online course as a preprogram student in a master's degree program. Her courses were offered through mail-out packages and WebBoard asynchronous conferencing courseware. Despite her experience of some of the courseware as inaccessible, she cited the advantages of asynchronous communication, formed valued friendships online, and described herself as "excited" about online learning.

Bernice

Bernice is a Canadian. She has a grown son and daughter and two grandchildren. Bernice is the secretary to her church council. She has been a college instructor for the past 21 years other than a 4-year period wherein she took a sojourn from teaching to accept a term as division chair of adult basic education. Bernice has a bachelor of art's degree with a major in French, a diploma in adult education and a master's degree in higher education.

Bernice weighed two-and-a-half pounds at birth, and is blind due to the condition of Retinopathy of Prematurity. She perceives it significant that she is "not a person who is newly adjusting to blindness." Bernice is a strong advocate for Braille literacy and is on the organizing committee for an upcoming conference bringing together professionals in that field. When asked about her philosophy on blindness, Bernice responded,

> I don't like a lot of the language attributed to blindness. Like, I don't like the term "disability" because it implies lack of ability and I don't consider myself to have a lack of ability. I don't like the word "impairment" because it's sort of—I think of impaired driving and such. That's kind of negative. But I don't have any alternate solutions to present either. I do consider myself a blind person, and I'm comfortable with that word, although I guess a lot of people with low vision aren't necessarily.... I'm comfortable with who I am. I get really frustrated about the negative connotations of blindness, particularly in a lot of hymns and as part of my religious affiliation.... I'm part of the school who considers myself an ordinary person who happens to be blind. And it's part of my identity and it's something that I shouldn't have to feel negative about.

Bernice is actively involved within the Canadian blindness system. She is on the Canadian National Institute for the Blind provincial division board and the national board. She is also on the Voice Print national board.

Bernice questions extremist views on inclusive education of blind children and adults. She herself went to a school for the blind for her first 10 years. She explained that because "it was the thing to do in the late sixties to have people go into regular schools," she went to the designated school for her neighborhood for Grades 11 and 12. When she identified the need for a program for the blind and people with low vision 21 years ago, and proposed starting the program at the college with whom she was employed, there was debate regarding the segregated nature of such a program. She explained, "this was kind of something that went against the grain to some degree because most people with disabilities were participating in the regular stream." She elaborated that she "wasn't against that," but wanted to pursue the program in any case because "I just felt that there might be a place for a program that would give people the coping skills and the confidence that they needed to go on to further education." The program currently has an enrollment of 44 students some of whom are international. The content emphasis is on Internet skills and

Microsoft applications, although Braille, English, and math are also taught.

Bernice has been working with computers since 1984, and her instructional capacity keeps her up-to-date with applications. She is able to train learners in the use of multiple adaptive technologies for people who are blind and low vision, and she herself primarily uses JAWS screen reading software. She does a great deal of research online, and some of her shopping online.

In a continuing effort to keep up-to-date and in consideration of online learning for the advancement of her own college program, Bernice enrolled in an online course titled "Barrier Free Online Learning for Students with Disabilities" instructed by Dr. Norman Coombs and Dick Banks of Equal Access to Software and Information (EASI) out of Rochester University. The course was delivered through the Blackboard learning moderation system. There were approximately 12 students in the course from Canada, the United States, and Russia. The course lasted 1 month with posted weekly lessons. Bernice described the course format and the process of engaging with it.

> So you went up and listened to the lesson and then there were links to different articles and different audio presentations that you could link to—they were right within the lesson. And that was really helpful because there were some things that kind of emphasized what was being explained in the lesson. And then at the end of the lesson there was an assignment.... There was an e-mail discussion list where we all shared our assignment and it was things like, "does your college or institution have a policy related to students with disabilities?" Or, accessible courseware design. Or, if your college has online courses what courseware are they using? And the object of the course was to come up with a presentation you could make to your faculty about designing accessible online courses.

The course design intentionally did not include use of a bulletin board. Bernice hesitated to comment on the functionality or accessibility of such a communication tool because she does not have direct experience with it, but when pressed, she described what she considers to be the drawback. She stated that bulletin boards

> are a pain, because you have to read all of the links before you get to the meat of the site. So using a LISTSERV or distribution list was much more effective than having to deal with Web-based interactive tools that are available through the Web course software.

The course primarily used e-mail for interaction. Bernice stated that the interaction between students and with the instructor was "very good." "The instructor was the moderator of the list essentially, and he would pick up on comments of the students and facilitate conversation of the e-mail list and that worked very well."

Through the course, and through a bonus presentation on accessible PowerPoint, Bernice experienced two other types of communication tools that she did not assess as functional. In the case of synchronous voice-based chat as administered through Chatterbox software, the problem was an issue of usability and not a result of sensory impairment. She explained,

> The biggest problem in using the Chat room was knowing when it was my turn to talk. You couldn't tell. You could hear other people talking. The idea was you had to hold the control key down and then talk, but if someone else was also doing the same thing, then I couldn't always figure out when it was my turn to talk and so I was a little hesitant.

The second attempted communication tool was an enhancement to the voice-based chat. Simultaneous with the chat, the instructor and students demonstrated PowerPoint slides. In order to access both the slide and the accompanying comments spontaneously as presented, Bernice would have had to be able to listen to both the spoken comments and the JAWS screen reading software vocalizing the slides simultaneously. This being impossible, Bernice elected to listen to the comments only and read the slides later.

Even with the two instances of communication tools that did not function optimally, Bernice assessed her experience of online learning as "very positive." She said, "It was fun! I loved it!" She attributed the positive nature of her experience largely to the consistent content and delivery. The online course content concerned how to make online courses accessible and thereby applied the teachings to the design. In addition, one of the course designers/instructors is blind and the other has low vision, thereby ensuring understanding of the frequently encountered barriers. As testament to her theory that other courses cannot be expected to be as accessible, Bernice was asked to validate and consult regarding the accessibility of three discrete online courses. Each of these was either entirely or largely incompatible with the JAWS screen reading software.

Bernice eloquently expressed the hopes of many blind people and the rationale for accessible education.

> Blind people in general do not want to have their needs met to the exclusion of people with vision because we're a very small percentage of the population. What we want (and maybe I shouldn't speak for all people, but what I think blind people and other people with disabilities want) is to be able to access the same educational material as anyone else would be able to access.

> And if there's a need for a neat visual thing, then that's okay. But there needs to be an alternate link available, an alternate description that describes what happened or what is going on in the class, or an alternate assignment, or audio presentation that includes the visual but describes what's going on interactively. I guess if multimedia is used it can be very powerful, and even for a blind person, as long as it doesn't exclude the person. As long as there is some way of including the person in the experience.

In summary of Bernice's story, she is a middle-aged Canadian who is actively involved in promoting quality of life for blind people. She uses JAWS screen reading software to access the computer, and is a college instructor training blind adults in the use of adaptive technologies to access the Internet and use Microsoft applications. She has a bachelor's and master's level degrees and completed a course titled "Barrier Free Online Learning" through Equal Access to Software and Information out of Rochester University. The course was delivered through the Blackboard learning moderation system. Even though she did not experience all of the communication tools as functional, Bernice was positive about the experience stating that it was "fun" and that she "loved it." She attributed the success of the experience largely to the informed and dedicated nature of the course designers/instructors.

Deborah

Deborah is a social justice advocate and has worked in this capacity since graduating with a bachelor's of psychology degree in 1978. She is currently employed providing training in technical assistance for Easter Seals Project Action that she described as "a grant funded through the Federal Transfer Administration to address issues of access and transportation for people with disabilities." Deborah was raised in the southern states and currently resides in Washington. She chose Washington both because of the national advocacy efforts providing opportunity for her contribution, and because of the number of options for transportation.

Both Deborah and her now 21-year-old daughter have a genetic condition called Retinoblastoma (cancer of the retina), although their experiences of the condition have been substantially different. Deborah has had no vision since she was 3 years old. Her daughter has some restricted vision, but with glasses is able to drive a car. Deborah described the condition and the circumstances within her life and her daughter's.

> It is something that once it is started, it is hereditary, or at least it is genetic so there's a chance that it will be inherited. But it always starts somewhere in the family and there is no traceable history of it in my family. So as far as I

> know, I'm the first one who's had it, so they didn't know to look for it. So it was only recognized as a problem when my mother began to notice spots in my eyes around the pupil that shouldn't be there and took me to an ophthalmologist and I was eighteen months old at the time. I went through what was the best process for treatment then, and their goal at that time really was not to have any hope of saving vision. They did hope to save one eye intact with the optic nerve in case any type of future research advances would make it possible to restore vision, but that was not possible so eventually they ended up having to remove both eyes. That occurred within the first three years. Retinoblastoma is a fairly well understood disease now, as it has gotten a lot of specific research out of St. Jude's hospital out of Memphis. And so they pretty much know that it's going to do what it's going to do over the first few years of life. And if you are able to control it, within a specific time period. My daughter has it. And she was treated at St. Jude's. We were prepared for it, so I had the ophthalmologist in the hospital when she was born to examine her. And at two weeks old we had her at St. Jude's hospital. And they did an excellent job. They saved both eyes.

While Deborah's daughter attended public school, Deborah herself attended a residential school for the blind. However, the school was in Deborah's home community so she attended there during the day but lived at home.

Deborah has been using computers for work since 1990. She considers herself "very proficient at what I use." This comprises a comprehensive list including Outlook, Internet Explorer, and numerous Microsoft applications such as Word, PowerPoint, and Excel. Deborah primarily uses JAWS screen reading software to access the computer.

Within a year or so of learning to use the computer, Deborah enrolled in an online course through Equal Access to Software and Information out of Rochester University, early in the organization's history, and early in the advent of online learning. It was a course designed to teach the Americans with Disabilities Act (ADA) requirements around employment. The course took place over a few months. Every 2 weeks until many of the 20 students lagged so far behind that the spacing of the lessons needed to be widened, one of approximately 10 lessons was distributed to each of the learners via e-mail. Deborah described the course design as a replication of a noninteractive traditional face-to-face classroom. "Basically, it was take a professor and have them write out everything that they would say in a lecture. They were very long lessons and they were very full—a lot of cut and paste from the regulations." The only other teaching strategy imposed was the case study. "They would have a particular case study where they would describe the scenario of a person with a disability, describe their job and how the ADA would apply in that particular situation." There was no interaction with the other students beyond an initial e-mail in which each learner briefly introduced him or herself.

When asked what it was like to be a blind online learner based on that particular experience, Deborah replied,

> That one was pretty painful.... The good thing about it was that it provided me with very quickly a great deal of information about Title One regulations and technical assistance guides. And it gave it to me in a very accessible format. But there was such a quantity of information. It was almost like if you've ever seen a technical assistance manual—it's huge—sent to me via e-mail over a period of months.... I ended up with a lot of information, but it was not a very accessible resource. It was easier to just have an electronic copy of the technical assistance manual.... I was excited about it at the time. It was a first online course I had ever taken. I was so glad it was going to be accessible. It was what I needed at the time.

Even though Deborah graciously described the positive elements of the course emphasizing the accessibility of the delivery and the importance of the content, she concluded her comment with the telling statement, "I have never sought to take such a course again."

While Deborah carefully assesses online offerings to determine whether they are text-intensive replications of a lecture hall, she is positive about the potential of online learning overall. She agreed to participate in the research in an effort to reflect and learn more about positive approaches to online learning. In terms of application, she is considering extending her career work through the provision of online learning, and personally is considering a graduate program online.

> From a personal standpoint, if I were to pursue additional education, I would certainly consider Web courses despite the things that I pointed out that I don't particularly like about them. Because it's easy. Because it's readily available. Because I can take that course and not have to worry about whether I can get to that campus at the certain time that I'm supposed to get to the campus. It gives you a certain amount of self-pacing and I really do like that because I'm a really intensive learner. So I'd just as soon work at my own pace, as opposed to waiting. So there are definitely advantages such as the convenience of sitting down in your own living room.

In summary of Deborah's story, she is a social justice advocate living in Washington. She is blind and primarily uses JAWS screen reading software to access the computer. She is computer proficient. Deborah's single experience of online learning, over 10 years ago, was not positive. The primary problem was a design that replicated a noninteractive lecture hall. She described the experience as "pretty painful." However, Deborah's perception of online learning has not been soured. She continues to explore online options both as a trainer and personally, as a means of enrolling in a master's degree program.

Shannon

Shannon is an outgoing, fun-loving woman with a sense of adventure. She described herself as always having been a "curious" person. "I like to know how things are, and why things are, and what things are." She loves to cook and to entertain.

Prior to high school, Shannon attended a state school for the blind, and then went to a public school. She graduated from university with a bachelor of arts degree with a major in recreation. Upon graduation, Shannon decided that she did not want to be "the kind of person" who lived in the shelter of one place for her entire life, so in her early 20s moved to Hawaii by herself. She worked in the restaurant business for "quite a while" and experienced discriminatory attitudes first-hand. She explained that she realized that "attitudes about people's disabilities was really the biggest barrier that many of us faced, and sometimes that could be our own attitudes about ourselves."

Inspired to make a difference in people's attitudes and the impact of those attitudes, Shannon started her own advocacy and action business in 1986 called "Open Access."

> And that's what I've been doing. Working with companies and working with people with disabilities. Mostly companies, and teaching them, when the ADA came out—the Americans with Disabilities Act, and really doing activities to get them to see how their own attitudes could either enhance or inhibit people's participation in employment, in getting services from a company, in participating in the community.

Shannon is a strong advocate for Braille literacy and believes that blind youth are doing themselves a grave injustice if they fail to learn to read and write Braille including functional use of a slate and stylus. However, having an adventurous spirit, Shannon has recently tried to expand her technological repertoire. Overall, the process has not been positive for Shannon.

> Okay, I got my first computer in 1999 and I will tell you, I got my first computer and like I am a techno-jinx! Everything I've gotten has either broken down within the first month (I promise I followed instructions), everything has had to go back to the shop and get re-thised and re-that so not only am I not only a jinx with the computer that my experience overall has not been a good experience. I mean, I just got a brand new Braille Note—I had to

> send it back to the shop because the dots were flying. They were coming up at wrong times. And the guy said, "You are the first person that had this on a brand new unit." I said, "naturally."

Shannon has mixed feelings regarding e-mail. She believes that people use it far too readily and make no other efforts to ensure that communication is accessible. She prefers the voice-to-voice connection of the telephone, but recognizes the advantages of e-mail in avoiding long distance charges. In addition, she stated, "sometimes e-mail is great to leave quick messages especially if you know people check it and you leave messages when they are sleeping." She believes that the Internet is a good resource and is therefore attempting to develop functional use of JAWS screen reading software. She said, "it is frustrating because a computer is designed for people who can see." She laughingly described taking 10 hours trying to compose a business letter layout and emerging only to ask for a manual typewriter.

In 2002 Shannon decided to challenge herself once again, attempting an online course registration in one of her passions—cooking. With the telephone in one hand, and the other hand on the keyboard, Shannon signed up for an online cooking class with Emeril Lagosse. She humorously described "trying to tab around up arrow, down arrow, put everything into a LISTSERV, doing all this other stuff." She said, "I got frustrated! I finally did get signed up but I got frustrated." She decided that if the online course enrollment was so entirely frustrating, that actually participating in the course could not be any better, so she elected not to take it. She said that she "bagged-out on the sign-in part."

The term Shannon used most frequently in contemplation of the possibility of online learning is "missing." She explained, "I kept thinking of all the things I was missing. I'm missing the smell of the food in this interchange. I realized I'm missing the cooking, and I love to cook." When asked whether she could imagine engaging in less tactile subjects online, such as pursuing a master's level degree Shannon replied that her style is to "evaluate each situation and circumstances." Her decision of whether to pursue face-to-face or online would depend on many factors such as "the class, circumstance, time of class, my time, and my computer skills." With reference to the course content, Shannon used the specific examples of "cooking online—No, a writing class online—Yes." However, overall, Shannon believes that face-to-face education is a better alternative. "I would be missing out on the sound of people's voices, the tones of their voices, the punctuation in their voices. I would be missing all that stuff." Further, she described her learning style as "learning through doing" and thereby believes that online learning "is not conducive to my learning mode."

In summary, Shannon is a social justice advocate who works in education and facilitating opportunities for Americans with disabilities. To date, she has primarily experienced the computer as frustrating and online learning as "missing." She successfully enrolled in an online cooking class and subsequently decided not to pursue the experience. She experienced the sign-up interface as frustrating, and did not feel that online would be an effective medium for delivering a cooking class. However, she recognizes the advantages of technologies such as e-mail and the World Wide Web, and the potential convenience of online learning. With regard to future enrollments, Shannon will assess opportunities based on the specific situation and circumstances.

Composing Stories

Now that you have read the seven stories, I would like to share what I was mindful of in writing them. This morning, I received a phone call from my mother. One of her many talents includes oil painting. She was asked to donate a painting and they asked that she include a life narrative on the back. She asked me to compose it. I think that the stories we write for interpretive empirical research are more like art bios than anything else. They are focussed sketches of multifaceted lives. I will include my Mom's bio to illustrate my point.

> Born and raised in the prairies of western Canada, Elaine Spitzer has cultured an aesthetic appreciation for nature and rural toil. She dedicated her career to teaching, specializing in music and reaching children who were academically struggling. After raising a son (a computer operating systems specialist) and a daughter (a professor), she and her husband retired to an acreage near Cochrane. They use Cochrane as their home base, from which they delight in visits with their five grandchildren, and enjoy their main hobby of birding, engaged in both locally and leading them to travel the world, to such destinations as Madagascar and Venezuela. Her hobbies inspire her oil painting. Elaine's favorites are paintings of birds, indigenous prairie flowers, and local highlights from her travels. She is a member of the Foothills Art Club.

The focus is on oil painting. The very first line begins with her "aesthetic appreciation." Appreciators of her paintings want to know why it is that she paints birds, barns, and adobe huts. But they also want to know more about Elaine. They want her fleshed out. They want her to live and breath, as much as she can across the back canvas of the painting they have been the highest bidder on through the silent auction. Likewise, the focus in each of the research narratives you have just read is on the experience of online learning, but in order to understand, it is helpful to know about their experience with computers, their life context, and the impact of blindness on their lives.

None of the narrative depictions prioritize blindness. In other words, the stories do not begin by describing the diagnostics of each participant, nor any other details associated with his or her being blind. This ordering parallels the self-presentation of the participants, as discussed below. People have multifaceted selves and blindness is only one surface of the prism. The participants did not emphasize blindness as an overshadowing or controlling domain in their lives, even though it was one of the criteria for research participation. One of my tasks as researcher was to determine what was one of the most meaningful facets to them personally. What did they share that was closest to the "I." I determined this by the frequency with which examples of this content were mentioned, the body language observed when it was discussed, the tone of voice, the emotion words used to describe the phenomena, and the point at which the participant offered the experience into the conversation. For example, was the phenomena brought up immediately after trust was established?

Madeline's important inner core is her family and her involvement with her sons while she was rearing them. Matthew emphasized his general life disposition of introspection, but also those who matter in his life. Martin's story begins by shockingly announcing his nine children, which holds even more intrigue when juxtaposed in the next lines with his multifaceted life filled with work and leisure pursuits. What is important to Sarah in the context of her family, is their education. She spoke not only of her own education, but what each of her husband and children had accomplished. Bernice's narrative reads like a balanced biography, the first paragraph sketching her family, work, volunteer contributions, and other pursuits. The presentation of Deborah's narrative presents a common example of the way in which we story our lives. If we choose a career with a strong identity, then we often describe ourselves by that role —"I *am* a social justice advocate." Also exemplified in the story of Deborah, people who are from tightly culturally bounded social groups by heritage tend to either self-identify, or be identified. In Deborah's case, her southern drawl and charming stories about her "sistahs" and how important it was to them that Deborah look acceptable is a core element. Finally, Shannon was presented differently than the others and Shannon was different from the others. In the final edits, I received some criticism that Shannon's story read trite compared to the others and I had to consider whether it required changing. The final judge was Shannon, and she like the others, was satisfied with the presentation. Unlike the others, the first lines do not present Shannon's roles, accomplishments, and relationships. Shannon is presented in personality and character.

Shannon is presented as "outgoing, fun-loving, with a sense of adventure," and this indeed captures her essence.

Seven Phenomenologies of Blind Online Learning

Considering the group of learners together, the demographics of these research participants are in keeping with what the literature tells us about online learners. Thompson (1998) wrote that online learners tend to be older than the traditional postsecondary student, married, employed full-time while studying, and female. All of the seven learners in this research were mature students. Six of the seven participants were currently, or had previously been married, or had children. Six of the seven participants were employed full-time while studying. Madeline was the only exception and she took on an accelerated course load. Five of the seven participants were female.

There were a variety of approaches to the delivery of the online courses. Madeline's, Deborah's, and Shannon's courses were delivered through Web sites and e-mail. Martin's and Bernice's courses were delivered through Blackboard courseware. Matthew's courses used First Class courseware. Sarah's courses used a WebBoard.

None of the courses were designed such that the learners could access them without using adaptive technologies. Madeline, Martin, Bernice, Deborah, and Shannon (each of whom is totally blind), and Sarah (who has low vision) primarily use JAWS screen reading software. In addition, Sarah uses a CCTV reader. Matthew primarily uses ZoomText enlarger software.

Deborah and Shannon did not have positive experiences with online learning. Deborah's dissatisfaction rested with the lack of course interactivity. However, she maintains positive perceptions of online learning, and is pursuing this avenue as a trainer, and potentially as a graduate student. Shannon's primary dissatisfaction was with the frustrating interface. She also described the experiential aspect of online learning as "missing"—missing conversations, and in the case of online cooking—smells and tastes.

Madeline, Matthew, Martin, Sarah, and Bernice had positive experiences of online learning. Each commented about the convenience of online learning, allowing them to study while maintaining family and/or work commitments. They also commented about the high level of online dialogue and sense of community as learners. Matthew described the experience as "fascinating," Martin as "liberating," Sarah as "really exciting," and Bernice as "fun," further stating that she "loved it!"

Madeline graduated from a program with a blended model (where the learners take most of their courses online, but meet together for annual concentrated-time study institutes). Matthew is currently enrolled in a program with a blended model. Matthew and Madeline were enthusiastic about this model and shared that they would not have it any other way. Martin's college offers some courses face-to-face and some online. Martin opts for the online delivery when available. Sarah has taken three courses toward a program that will occur entirely online. To date, Bernice has taken only one online course, but an entire online certificate is available should she wish to pursue it.

While five of the learners were positive about their experience, none of the learners can be classified as what Boshier and Mun Onn (2000) would call "techno-utopians." In other words, these learners do not believe that online learning is the educational panacea. Most commented about the necessary initiation of young adults through a face-to-face postsecondary experience. Madeline's occasional struggle with motivation in online courses surprised even herself. Both Matthew and Martin stated that if they were not working full-time they would have opted for face-to-face education. Bernice doubts the accessibility of most online experiences, and largely attributes her success to the intentional accessible design of the course and its informed instructors.

In terms of accessibility, with one exception, none of the courses were universally designed and each had instances of poor functionality and/or incompatibility with adaptive technologies such as screen reading software. The only exception was Deborah's course that was completely accessible, but also completely noninteractive. Madeline reported that her instructor attempted implementation of a bulletin board and that neither Madeline nor her sighted student colleagues experienced it as functional. Matthew could not follow the synchronous text-based chat with his capacity to read only a few words at a time, and the rapidity with which the lines scrolled up and thus out of his focus. Martin could not access the synchronous text-based chat at all. It was seemingly incompatible with the JAWS screen reading software. Sarah could not access the bulletin board postings independently. She relied on her husband to read them out to her. Bernice found it challenging to participate in the synchronous voice-based chat and impossible to listen to the same-time screen reader translation of the PowerPoint slides and the accompanying translation. The initial interface of Shannon's course was so frustrating that she did not pursue the learning experience. Three of these instances of inaccessibility or incompatibility are unique to learners with sensory impairments. A strong case can be made for widespread applicability beyond a disability issue of the other four instances.

Shannon withdrew from the learning experience. Notably, she had neither of the conditions supporting the others' online learning experiences. Martin, Bernice, and Deborah are experienced computer users and might be considered technologically proficient. Madeline, Matthew, and Sarah have regular access to human technological assistance—the women through their spouses, and Matthew through his work.

Chapter 5 Conclusion

This chapter presented an account of the online learning experiences of seven blind online learners. Each informant's story was presented individually. The seven stories were then interwoven. Commonalities and discrepancies were considered to inform what it is like to be a blind online learner. The next chapter, chapter 6, presents an interpretive dimension of reflexive analysis. The three research questions form the pillars of this chapter. What it is like to be a blind online learner is further informed by considering the themes emerging in the interviews and then analyzing these themes in relationship. For example, this chapter presented the overall experiences of five of the learners as positive and two as negative. What other factors, such as computer proficiency, accessibility, and interactive course design might have informed the learners' overall evaluation of their experience? The second research question regarding the best design of online courses is informed by Coombs and Banks (2000) 16 tips for the design and facilitation of online courses. Which of these tips were corroborated within the informants' depictions of their experience? Finally, the interview transcripts were revisited to highlight what the informants expressed in answer to the third research question regarding the impact of online learning of blind adults.

CHAPTER 6

INTERPRETIVE RESEARCH ANALYSIS

INTRODUCTION

As the first stage of the reflexive analysis, chapter 5 told the stories of seven blind online learners. These stories were written in accordance with the phenomenological tradition. van Manen (1997) explained that phenomenology seeks to address what matters. With respect to this research, the inquiry concerns what matters in the experience of online learning for blind adults. van Manen wrote, "phenomenology must describe what is given to us in immediate experience without being obstructed by pre-conceptions and theoretical notions" (p. 184). In chapter 5 the stories of the seven informants were told on their terms. Where the meaning might have been interpreted ambiguously, their words were directly quoted. Where clarity and consistency in presentation might be gained through paraphrasing, the accounts were authored by the researcher. All of the stories were validated by the informants. All of their requests for edits were respected.

This chapter, dedicated to the second stage of the analysis, applies the three questions guiding the inquiry to interpret those stories. Interpretation differs from analysis of traditional research in three main ways. First,

Seeing Beyond Blindness, 97–146

the experience and its discourse are not considered objective. The phenomenon is a story. While this is not to say it is fictive, the words chosen to story the experience in part construct that experience. Second, the story is constructed by the participants. The open questions provide a space for the informants to reflect and for the story to emerge as fits each participant. The researcher does not pre-construct categories or deductively interrogate. Third, variance is recognized both between and within stories. The participant is not forced to select and thereby reject binary or mutually exclusive categories. Martin, for example, expressed that he experienced interaction throughout his online courses, and yet generally questions the idea of interactivity within online learning. Such dialectical issues with their inherent ambiguity are not ignored, stifled, or resolved within reflexive research.

The first question within this research asks what it is like to be a blind online learner. The question derives from hermeneutics (Gadamer, 1999). van Manen (1997) defined hermeneutics as "the theory and practice of interpretation" (p. 179). He further explained that the word's origin is in Greek mythology. The Greek god Hermes' role was "to communicate messages from Zeus and other gods to the ordinary mortals" (p. 179). van Manen wrote that hermeneutics is "necessary when there is possibility for misunderstanding" (p. 179). With respect to this research, there is possibility for misunderstanding regarding attitudes about blindness, the evolution of online learning, and the role of technology in the lives of blind adults. One of the goals of this inquiry is therefore to move outwards from the direct accounts of the seven learners, penetrating through the shared cultural meanings of blindness, technology, and online learning to interpret what is meaningful about blind online learning.

The approach to interpretation adopted within this research is consistent with what Aspland (1999) called a methodological pastiche. Inquiring into what it is like to be a blind online learner draws upon phenomenology in that the informants were asked to describe their "lived experience" in online courses (van Manen, 1997, p. 180). The analysis moves outside phenomenology in that it addresses the resonance between the theories as presented in the literature and the experiences of the learners. Questioning what it is like to be a blind online learner derives directly out of hermeneutics. Yet, the analysis moves outside of hermeneutics in that the project has pragmatic goals. The inquiry has the pragmatic goals of: (a) informing blind adults as to whether online learning is an educational avenue worth consideration, and if so, how best to participate as an online learner, and (b) educating instructors and course designers regarding best practices in online learning, particularly for blind students.

Each of the seven online learners had a unique experience of online learning. The courses for six of the learners were offered through five different postsecondary institutions. Two learners enrolled in courses through the same organization, but with approximately a 10-year span between the course offerings meaning substantially different course design. The seventh learner enrolled in a course through private industry.

Among the diversity, there are commonalities uniting the experiences of the learners. The participants can be grouped according to: (a) use of adaptive technologies, (b) experience of course accessibility, (c) experience of course design including use of communication tools, (d) evaluative perceptions of the experience, (e) eye condition, (f) experience of interactivity, (g) nationality (Americans and Canadians), (h) self-efficacious beliefs, and (i) technological proficiency and/or regular access to human supports. Interpretation of the experiences of the seven blind online learners was facilitated through constructing a series of grids matching varying combinations of the experiential factors. The section of the chapter addressing the first research question—what is it like to be a blind online learner—thereby poses questions such as: (a) did the use of adaptive technologies promote course accessibility, and (b) did those who experienced accessibility within their courses evaluate their courses as positive overall.

Interpretation of the second research question regarding recommended design characteristics is conducted in accordance with the literature. The stories resonate with the 16 tips for online learning as composed by Coombs and Banks (2000). The accordance of the experiences of the participants with these tips was at times surprising. Prior to being privileged to the stories of the seven blind online learners, the tip to use e-mail as the communication tool of choice rather than asynchronous bulletin boards or synchronous voice or text chats seemed counterintuitive. It seemed unlikely that e-mail could foster the desired level of interaction and critical thinking. However, the evidence provided by the participants in favor of e-mail is compelling.

The third guiding research question queries the impact of blind adults studying online. Data on impact is interpreted in two ways: (a) through identification of themes emerging from the stories, and (b) validating themes as emerging from the literature through direct probing within the interviews. Categories emerging from the interactive interviews included: (a) impact on the attitudes of fellow students and resulting social action; (b) alteration of the design of online courses reportedly benefiting all of the learners, not just those who are blind; and (c) the learners' advancement of transferable computing skills. Two themes were identified through the literature and posed to the research participants in the form of questions. First, will online learning become the new type of segregated education for blind adults? Second, are blind online learners sacrificing an ambassadorial role and thereby impacting public attitudes in deleterious ways?

What it is Like to be a Blind Online Learner

The first question guiding the research is—what is it like to be a blind online learner. Through identifying and then examining the relationships between themes, one can query what the experiences of these seven participants reveal about blind online learners more generally. A metaphorical geological vein meandering through the mass of data is that what applies to blind online learners usually encompasses online learners more generally. The goal of this section of the chapter, then, is to reflect outwards from the stories of the seven blind online learners to comment on what it is like to be a blind online learner, and what it is like to be an online learner generally, without specifying the characteristic of blindness.

Nine thematic categories emerged from two sources: (a) directly through conversation with the research participants; and (b) through the literature and through online discussion, provoking interview probes. The themes are presented in alphabetical order of the main conceptual words.

Category One—(use of) Adaptive Technologies

All of the participants used adaptive technologies to access information and communications through their computers and to facilitate output. Six of the seven participants (Madeline, Martin, Sarah, Bernice, Deborah, and Shannon) primarily used various versions of JAWS screen reading software. Matthew was the exception. He used ZoomText screen enlarging software and a handheld magnifier. Madeline, Martin, Bernice, and Deborah used a Braille embosser. Madeline, Martin, Bernice, Deborah, and Shannon used a handheld Braille device with a refreshable display. Sarah used a CCTV reader for print-based materials.

Category Two—(Experience of) Course Accessibility

For the purposes of this research, a course component was considered accessible if it was experienced as compatible with the participants' chosen adaptive technology such that they could fully receive and process the information and/or use the interactive communication tools in a timely matter. Madeline experienced the digital content modules, the e-mail, and the LISTSERV as accessible. She experienced the printed texts and the bulletin board as inaccessible. Matthew experienced the digital content modules, the e-mail, the LISTSERV, the printed texts and the bulletin board as accessible. He experienced the synchronous text-based chat as inaccessible. Martin experienced the digital content modules, the e-mail, the LISTSERV and the bulletin board as accessible. He experienced the printed texts and synchronous text-based chat as inaccessible. Sarah experienced the digital content modules, the e-mail, and the LISTSERV as accessible. She experienced the printed texts and the bulletin board as inaccessible. Bernice experienced the digital content modules, the e-mail, and the LISTSERV as accessible. She experienced synchronous voice-based chat and simultaneous slide show presentation and voice discussion as inaccessible. Deborah experienced the digital content modules, the e-mail and the LISTSERV as accessible. She did not experience any inaccessible components. Shannon experienced the sign-in process as inaccessible, and thereby discontinued the experience.

The participants' experiences of accessibility and inaccessibility of the course components are summarized in Table 6.1 The symbol A indicates accessibility, I indicates inaccessibility, and N/A indicates that the component was not part of the course design.

In summary of the experiences of accessibility of the blind online learners, Shannon's experiences are not included because she discontinued her involvement immediately following course enrolment. All six of the included participants experienced digital content modules and all six found them to be accessible. Three of the four participants who experienced printed texts found them to be inaccessible, and one experienced accessibility. All six of the participants who used e-mail experi-

Table 6.1. (In)accessibility of Course Components

Participants	*Digital Content Module*	*Printed Text*	*E-mail*	*LIST-SERV*	*Bulletin Board*	*Synchronous Text-Based Chat*	*Synchronous Voice Chat*	*Simultaneous Slide and Voice*
Madeline	A	I	A	A	I	N/A	N/A	N/A
Matthew	A	A	A	A	A	I	N/A	N/A
Martin	A	I	A	A	A	I	N/A	N/A
Sarah	A	I	A	A	I	N/A	N/A	N/A
Bernice	A	N/A	A	A	N/A	N/A	I	I
Deborah	A	N/A	A	A	N/A	N/A	N/A	N/A
Shannon	N/A	N/A	N/A	N/A	N/A	N/A	N/A	N/A

enced it as an accessible communication tool. All six participants also used a class LISTSERV within the e-mail communication tool and experienced it as accessible. Experience of the bulletin board was split with two participants experiencing it as accessible, and two as inaccessible. The two participants who experienced text-based chat experienced it as inaccessible, and the one who used voice-based chat also experienced it as inaccessible. Finally, the one participant who experienced simultaneous slideshow presentation and voice discussion found it to be inaccessible.

Category Three—Course Design

As recorded above, two types of information distribution media and six types of communication tools were experienced across the courses of the seven online learners. Shannon's experience is excluded from this presentation because she did not participate in the online course and thus could not comment on the course design. All six participants experienced digital content modules. Four received printed texts. All six used e-mail and communications via LISTSERV. Four used a bulletin board. Two experienced synchronous text-based chat. One used synchronous voice-based chat. One experienced a simultaneous slideshow presentation and voice discussion.

Across the six participants, three experienced courses delivered through Web sites, all of which also included e-mail and one of which also included a WebBoard. Madeline's courses and Deborah's course were delivered through Web sites and e-mail. Sarah's courses were delivered through Web sites, e-mail and WebBoards. Three of the courses were delivered using learning moderation systems. Matthew's courses were delivered through the First Class learning moderation system. Martin's courses and Bernice's course were delivered through the BlackBoard learning moderation system. Of the experienced learning moderation systems, BlackBoard was the most frequently experienced.

The other varying design characteristic concerned whether the courses were delivered through a pure online model or whether the program was designed according to a model whereby the learners had both face-to-face and online courses. Of the six participants who completed (an) online course(s), three programs were delivered both online and face-to-face and three designed to be entirely online. Madeline and Matthew participated in a blended model, which for the purposes of this research, is defined as a model whereby a cohort of students meets face-to-face for one or more concentrated-time study institutes and takes the majority of their courses online. Martin enrolled in both face-to-face and online courses within his program, but not through an intentionally blended model. Martin's university is creating online counterparts to many of their face-to-face courses. Martin enrolls in the online courses as they are made available. He enrolls in face-to-face courses when the online alternative has not yet been developed. Sarah is participating in an entirely online program. Bernice and Deborah have each completed one course. Should they decide to pursue further courses through the same program, the courses they completed each count toward one unit in an entirely online certificate program.

Category Four—Evaluative Perceptions of the Experience

This category depicts the overall evaluative perception of the experience. Five of the seven participants experienced online learning positively. The remaining two experienced it negatively. Of the five who experienced it positively: (a) Madeline described it as more positive than negative, (b) Matthew described it as fascinating, (c) Martin described it as liberating, (d) Sarah described it as really exciting, and (e) Bernice described it as fun and further commented that she loved it. Of the two who experienced it negatively: (a) Deborah described it as pretty painful, and (b) Shannon described it as missing.

Category Five—Eye Condition

Criteria for participation included that the participants be blind and use adaptive technologies to access the computer. In the first instance, blindness as defined in North America means that individuals are either without vision or have substantially impaired vision. In the second instance, use of adaptive technologies was included as a criterion so that research participation would be meaningful. It is conceivable that someone could have low vision such that they are classified as legally blind, but have vision to the degree that their use of a computer and thereby participation in online learning is no different than that of a sighted person.

Five of the participants in this research (Madeline, Martin, Bernice, Deborah, and Shannon) have no sight. Four of these individuals have been totally blind since shortly after birth and one (Deborah) since she was 3 years old. The other two individuals have low vision. Matthew has had low vision since early childhood. Sarah has had low vision for the past 16 years.

Category Six—(Experience of) Interactivity

As defined within this research, interactivity means that there is meaningful two-way communication between the instructor and students and between the students of the course. This includes an iterative feedback loop whereby correspondence takes into account previous messages and builds on or counters these postings. Shannon attempted to acquire interaction by phoning the organization offering the online cooking course and propping the phone between her shoulder and ear while she used her hands to operate the keyboard. As described within Shannon's story in chapter 5, the interface was so frustrating that even this attempted interaction resulted in discontinuation.

Of the six other participants who completed (an) online course(s), five experienced the course(s) as interactive. Deborah did not experience the online course as interactive. While the e-mail communication tool was used, it did not facilitate interaction. E-mail was used for an initial introduction of the course participants. Beyond that first instance, it was used for one-way distribution of information from the instructors, and one-way submission of assignments from the students.

Category Seven—Nationality

Of the seven research participants, four are Canadians. Madeline and Bernice reside in British Columbia. Matthew and Sarah reside in Alberta. Three of the four Canadians enrolled in courses through a Canadian institution. Bernice completed a course offered out of a postsecondary institution in the United States. Three of the seven research participants are Americans. Martin resides in Iowa. Deborah resides in Washington, DC. Shannon resides in Hawaii. All three enrolled in courses out of the United States of America.

Category Eight—Self-Efficacious Beliefs

Consideration of the role of self-efficacy in the experiences of blind online learners emerged from an online correspondent who is researching this psychological construct. Self-efficacy is the belief that one can successfully accomplish a specific goal or task. Psychological studies, such as those involving athletes, have linked self-efficacy and performance, often showing a positive correlation. Madeline, Matthew, Martin, Sarah, Bernice, and Deborah all retrospectively self-reported positive efficacious beliefs about their abilities to succeed in online courses. In addition, all of them expressed generalized feelings of self-efficacy. Sarah said, "I think you can do practically anything you set your mind to. Except maybe drive a car—you know the obvious things that you really do need vision for." In other words, belief that they could succeed was not confined to the instance of the online course. Deborah shared, "I don't often stop to consider whether I can do something, especially as a BLIND person, my consideration is HOW I'm going to do it." They each had a history of experiences that required extra effort or problem-solving beyond that of a sighted individual. Within the context of education, Bernice explained, "Learning as a blind person is often challenging. You often have to be able to think of coping strategies that other people often don't think about. You have to be assertive to make your needs known." These experiences of conquering challenges appeared to have given them a generalized belief in their ability to succeed.

The only exception in the area of self-efficacy regarding online learning was Shannon. Shannon demonstrated a generalized positive self-esteem. She expressed that she had succeeded in moving many states away on her own when she graduated with a bachelor's degree and in subsequently setting-up and running her own business. She reported incidents in which other women commented on her achievements, noting that they had not accomplished nearly to the same degree and yet they were sighted. However, in the realm of computers, Shannon's experience has shaken her confidence. When asked whether or not she felt that she could succeed in the online course prior to enrolling, she answered,

> I didn't believe or disbelieve. I didn't know. Like I do everything else. I just figured, "Oh well, hell, I'll try." So, I tried to sign up and then I went, "Oh hell!" Got frustrated.... I don't have a low frustration point. I'm a person that's like, "Okay, I'll keep trying. I'll get this. I'll get this." But I seem to have a lower frustration rate with the computer.

Category Nine—Technological Proficiency and/or the Existence of Human Supports

Three of the seven research participants rated themselves as technologically proficient. Martin and Bernice are responsible for training others in the use of technology. Deborah uses computers extensively within her job and has been using them for over 10 years. Four of the participants did not rate themselves as technologically proficient. Three of the four stated that they are competent at the computer-related tasks that they perform on a regular basis. These three, Madeline, Matthew, and Sarah, also have regular access to human technological supports. Madeline and Sarah both have technologically proficient spouses who assist them on a regular basis. Matthew works in close proximity to his former place of employment where he developed a friendship with a colleague in computing services. As the fourth participant who does not consider herself computer proficient, Shannon is the only participant who does not have regular access to human technological supports.

Relationship Between (use of) Adaptive Technologies and Course Accessibility

Nine factors emerging as salient in the experience of being a blind online learner are described above. The goal of the next section of the chapter is to interpret factors in combination to determine whether relationships can be posed between them. The first queried relationship is between the first category that explores the participants' use of adaptive technologies with the second category examining course accessibility. The relationship is posed to ask whether the types of adaptive technologies used by the seven research participants made a difference in their experience of course component accessibility. This question is explored in Table 6.2. For the purposes of this analysis, only course components experienced by two or more participants were included. Printed text was also not included because it is not accessed through adaptive technologies. The numerator in each cell represents the number of participants for whom the component was accessible. The denominator represents the overall number of participants who experienced this course component.

Notably there is only one participant who primarily uses ZoomText screen enlarging software, whereas the other five participants primarily use JAWS screen reading software. The relationship between the use of adaptive technologies and course accessibility can therefore only hint at questions that might be further pursued. There appears to be no discrepancy between learners using ZoomText and learners using JAWS in terms

Table 6.2. Relationship Between Use of Adaptive Technologies and Course Accessibility

Participants	*Digital Content Module*	*E-mail*	*LIST-SERV*	*Bullentin Board*	*Sychronous Text Chat*
Online Leaners Using JAWS (n = 5)					
Using JAWS	5/5	5/5	5/5	1/3	0/1
Online Learners Using ZoomText (n = 1)					
Using ZoomText	1/1	1/1	1/1	1/1	0/1

of accessing digital content modules, e-mail, LISTSERVs and text-based chat. The first three components were unanimously accessed by users of both types of software. The final component was experienced as inaccessible by both the user of ZoomText and the user of JAWS. A relationship between accessibility and adaptive technologies might be explored with respect to the bulletin board course component. Three participants using JAWS attempted use of the bulletin board and only one experienced it as accessible. The inaccessibility of the bulletin board when one cannot see the screen is intuitive due to two design characteristics of this communication tool: (a) read and unread messages are identified by color or icon (such as a flag), and (b) individual messages are not clearly tagged as discrete and require visual cues such as the open space between lines of text for separation. Matthew, the online learner who was able to see the screen using ZoomText screen enlarging software, experienced the bulletin board interface as accessible.

Relationship Between Course Accessibility and Technological Proficiency

The next table presents an inquiry into whether the participants' self-assessed technological proficiency and/or regular access to human supports appeared to influence whether or not they experienced course components as accessible. Table 6.3 plots accessibility of course components against three categorizations: (a) self-assessment as technologically proficient, (b) self-assessment as not technologically proficient with regular access to human supports, and (c) self-assessment as technologically proficient with no access to human supports. This final category is included in the chart to make the condition salient for reflection. However, Shannon's decision to withdraw prior to experiencing the course means that this category within the factor of technological proficiency cannot be plotted against accessibility of course components. The printed text course component is not included in this analysis because of the nonsensical nature of comparing the noncomputer medium of printed text with technological proficiency in the domain of computers. The numerator in each cell is the number of participants who experienced the course component as accessible and the denominator is the number of participants who experienced the course component.

There is no distinction between the two represented groups (those who self-assess as technologically proficient and those who self-assess as not technologically proficient but have regular access to human supports) with respect to the three seemingly accessible technologies of digital content modules, e-mail, and the LISTSERV. One of each of the participants

Table 6.3. Relationship Between Course Accessibility and Technological Proficiency

Participants	*Digital Content Mocule*	*E-mail*	*LIST-SERV*	*Bulletin Board*	*Synchronous Text-Based Chat*	*Synchronous Voice Chat*	*Simultaneous Slide and Voice*
Participants who self-assessed as technologically proficient (n = 3)	3/3	3/3	3/3	1/1	0/1	0/1	0/1
Participants who self-assessed as not technologically proficient with regular access to human supports (n = 3)	3/3	3/3	3/3	1/3	0/1	0/0	0/0
Participants who self-assessed as not technologically proficient without regular access to human supports (n = 1)	0/0	0/0	0/0	0/0	0/0	0/0	0/0

in the two technological proficiency groups experienced synchronous text-based chat and both found it inaccessible. Only one participant experienced synchronous voice-based chat and simultaneous slideshow presentation and voice discussion, yielding no one for comparison in the not technologically proficient category.

The one course component that proves interesting for comparison between the two groups is the bulletin board. The one participant who self-assessed as technologically proficient and used the bulletin board (Martin) found it accessible. Two of the three participants who self-assessed themselves as not technologically proficient, with regular access to human supports, experienced the bulletin board as inaccessible. The two women (Madeline and Sarah) shared that they rely on their husbands to support them in the use of higher-level computer tasks. Madeline tried the bulletin board and said that she could not get it to work, and was relieved when the instructor reverted to e-mail. Elsewhere within the interview, she commented that she feels that she has not become as computer savvy as she might be because she assesses it unnecessary to devote the time to this development given that her husband is a senior systems analyst. Sarah said that she cannot get her screen reading software to identify which messages are read or unread, or to navigate discrete entries. She awaits her husband's return from work and he reads the unread bulletin board postings out to her. Charting the relationship between self-assessed technological proficiency and related access to human supports against experienced accessibility of course components indicates that the following hypothesis warrants further exploration—adults who are not technologically proficient who have regular access to human supports might develop their skills to a lesser extent and might thereby experience more of the course components as inaccessible.

Relationship Between Self-Efficacious Beliefs and Technological Proficiency

An online correspondent is researching the relationship between self-efficacious beliefs and the various learning moderation systems used to design and deliver online courses. This relationship does not warrant further exploration within this research because interest in, or appreciation for, the relevance of learning moderation systems did not emerge in the interviews. In other words, learning moderation systems was almost a nontopic as far as the research participants were concerned.

What does warrant further analysis is the relationship between self-efficacious beliefs and technological proficiency. Examination of this relationship does not require charting. Six of the seven participants reported feeling self-efficacious about completing an online course. Shannon, as the exception, said that she thought that maybe she would succeed and maybe she would not. Shannon successfully enrolled in the course midst a great deal of frustration, and then withdrew. Shannon's interview transcripts indicate that her prior experience with computer technologies and resultant feelings may have impacted her ambivalent feelings about whether or not she could succeed prior to enrolling in the online cooking course. She is one of the four individuals who self-assessed herself as not being technologically proficient. She differed from the other three in that they had regular access to human supports. The multi-dimensional relationship that warrants further inquiry then is that between self-assessment as not technologically proficient, not having regular access to human supports, not having self-efficacious beliefs about participating in online learning, and not succeeding in the course.

Evaluative Perception Domain

The next series of relationships are between the evaluative perceptions of the experience and eight categories of the participants' demographics or components of their experience. The seven relationships to be considered include those between the evaluative perceptions of online learning and: (a) course accessibility, (b) course design including the use of communication tools, (c) eye condition, (d) interactivity, (e) nationality, (f) self-efficacious beliefs, (g) technological proficiency and/or the existence of human supports, and (h) gender. Examination of the relationship between the evaluative perceptions of the experience and the use of adaptive technologies is not possible within the current research. There is no basis for comparison. Six of the participants use JAWS screen reading software. Matthew is the only exception, in that he uses ZoomText screen enlarging software. Matthew evaluated the online experience positively, but within his story did not attribute this evaluation to the use of ZoomText to access the course. The purpose of this exploration is to determine factors that might contribute to the perceived success or failure of online learning.

Relationship Between Evaluative Perceptions of the Experience and Course Accessibility

Table 6.4 presents the relationship between the evaluative perceptions of the experience and course accessibility. The numerator in each cell represents the number of participants who experienced the course component as accessible, and the denominator represents the number of participants who used that course component.

Accessibility does not appear to have been a major factor in the relative evaluation of online learning. This is indicated by both the charted relationship and Deborah's comments. Deborah and Shannon are the two participants who evaluated the experience of online learning negatively. Shannon withdrew prior to experiencing any of the course components. Deborah experienced digital content modules, e-mail and a LISTSERV. She indicated experiencing each of these as accessible, yet she evaluated the course negatively. She commented that accessibility was not the problem, and in fact was one of the positive components of the course. It must be noted that all of the informants, with the exception of Shannon who did not participate in the actual course, experienced the digital content modules and e-mail as accessible. In other words, they were able to access the course content and communicate within the course. Even though each of the participants with the exception of Shannon experienced inaccessibility of course components, the minimum accessibility requirements were met. They were able to be participants in the courses. The nonemerging relationship between the evaluative perception of online learning and accessibility indicates that making an online course accessible is not enough to make it a positive experience, or in other words, accessibility is necessary but not sufficient.

Relationship Between the Evaluative Perception of Online Learning and the Course Design

Two aspects of course design were considered with reference to the evaluative perceptions of online learning. It was queried whether participants who experienced a blended model were more likely to evaluate their experience positively than participants who studied purely online, and whether enrolling in courses delivered through Web sites versus through learning moderation systems appeared to have had an impact on evaluative perceptions. Tables 6.5 and 6.6 chart the factors of evaluative perceptions of online learning and: (a) program model, and (b) course delivery. The number in each cell represents the number of participants who experienced each type of course design. The numbers do not add up to the number of participants because Shannon cannot be counted into the course design element.

There is no strong evidence to predict a relationship between the evaluative perception of online learning and either the program model or the course delivery with respect to whether or not the course was

Table 6.4. Relationship Between Evaluative Perceptions of the Experience and Course Accessibility

Evaluation	*Digital Content Module*	*Printed Text*	*E-mail*	*LIST-SERV*	*Bulletin Board*	*Synchronous Test-BasedChat*	*Synchronous Voice Chat*	*Simultaneous Slide and Voice*
Evaluated the experience of online learning positively ($n = 5$)	5/5	1/4	5/5	5/5	2/4	0/2	0/1	0/1
Evaluated the experience of online learning negatively ($n = 2$)	1/1	0/0	1/1	1/1	0/0	0/0	0/0	0/0

Table 6.5. Relationship Between the Evaluative Perception of Online Learning and the Program Model

Evaluation	*Experienced a Blended Model (Online Learning and Face-to-face)*	*Experienced a Pure Online Model*
Evaluated the experience of online learning positively ($n = 5$)	3	2
Evaluated the experience of online learning negatively ($n = 2$)	0	1

Table 6.6. Relationship Between the Evaluative Perception of Online Learning and Course Delivery (With Respect to Learning Moderation Systems)

Evaluation	*Courses Delivered Through a Learning Moderation System*	*Courses Delivered Through Web Sites and one or More Communicaion Tools*
Evaluated the experience of online learning positively ($n = 5$)	2	3
Evaluated the experience of online learning negatively ($n = 2$)	1	0

delivered through a learning moderation system. With respect to the first factor, the participants in the blended model, particularly those with concentrated-time study institutes and the majority of courses online were much more vocal about the positive nature of this model, than were the participants in the purely online model. However, two out of the three participants in the purely online model were also positive about the online learning experience, and did not posit any criticisms of the model. Deborah, as the participant in the purely online model who evaluated her overall experience as negative, did not mention the purely online model as a factor in her discontent. It must be noted that Deborah took only one course toward what may be a unit toward a certificate offered through a purely online model, and at the time of Deborah's enrollment the course was stand-alone in that the certificate was not yet developed.

In terms of the course delivery with respect to whether or not the course was delivered using a learning moderation system, there once again appears to be no relationship with the evaluative perception of the course. The learning moderation system was not an unprompted category emerging out of the comments of the informants. In all cases, the learning moderation system, or lack-thereof, was not mentioned until probed by the researcher. Within the interactive interviews, learning moderation systems appeared to be a null-and-void category. Interestingly, the researcher had to define learning moderation system and describe courseware for those whose courses were designed using Web sites and one or more communication tools, as they did not appear aware that such courseware packages existed.

Relationship Between Evaluative Perception of Online Learning and Eye Condition

The relationship between the evaluative perception of online learning and legally blind (low vision) versus totally blind are considered in Table 6.7 to query whether there is more likelihood for learners to evaluate online learning as positive if they have some vision versus if they have no vision.

A relationship between extent of vision and evaluative perception of online learning did not emerge through the interviews. The two participants who evaluated the experience of online learning as negative have no vision. However, this appears to be coincidental and not predictive, as the other three participants who have no vision evaluated online learning positively.

Table 6.7. Relationship Between the Evaluative Perception of Online Learning and Eye Condition

Evaluation	*Participants who Have no Vision*	*Participants who Have low Vision*
Evaluated the experience of online learning positively (n = 5)	3	2
Evaluated the experience of online learning negatively (n = 2)	2	0

Relationship Between Evaluative Perception of Online Learning and Interactivity

The overall evaluative perception of online learning was considered with respect to the participants' depictions of the online courses as interactive or noninteractive and shown in Table 6.8. The question is whether learners who describe the experience as noninteractive are more likely to evaluate the overall experience of online learning negatively.

The perceptions of the seven research participants indicate that there may be a relationship between course interactivity and overall evaluation of online learning. The five participants who described their course(s) as interactive unanimously evaluated the experience of online learning positively. The two participants who described the experience as noninteractive both evaluated the experience of online learning negatively. Even though Shannon attempted an interactive experience of course enrollment by using the computer and telephone simultaneously, it remained noninteractive and the frustration led her to withdraw from the course prior to engaging. Deborah completed the course, but described the experience as unsatisfactory because there was no give-and-take with the instructors and no relationship with the other learners.

Relationship Between the Evaluative Perception of Online Learning and Nationality

In order to query whether citizens of the United States of America or Canada are likely to be unified in their evaluative perception of online learning, nationality, and evaluative perceptions of online learning were considered and charted in Table 6.9.

The four Canadians evaluated online learning positively. Of the Canadians, Bernice completed her course through the Rochester Institute of Technology, an American institution. Of the two Americans who com-

Table 6.8. Relationship Between the Evaluative Perception of Online Learning and Interactivity

Evaluation	*Participants who Described the Online Course(s) as Interactive*	*Participants who Described the Online Course(s) as not Interactive*
Evaluated the experience of online learning positively ($n = 5$)	5	0
Evaluated the experience of online learning negatively ($n = 2$)	0	2

Table 6.9. Relationship Between the Evaluative Perception of Online Learning and Nationality

Evaluation	*Participants Residing in Canada*	*Participants Residing in the U.S.A*
Evaluated the experience of online learning positively ($n = 5$)	4	1
Evaluated the experience of online learning negatively ($n = 2$)	0	1

pleted their courses, one evaluated online learning positively and the other negatively. There is no suggestion of a relationship between nationality and overall evaluative perceptions of online learning in this research.

Relationship Between the Evaluative Perception of Online Learning and Self-Efficacious Beliefs

Table 6.10 considers the evaluative perception of online learning with respect to the participants' self-efficacious beliefs about online learning. The question is asked whether those who believe that they can succeed in online learning are more likely to evaluate the experience positively than those who are less certain of their success. Discussed above was the idea that the multidimensional relationship between self-assessment as not technologically proficient, not having regular access to human supports, not having self-efficacious beliefs about participating in online learning, and not succeeding in the course warrants further research. This section adds another layer to the inquiry, asking if these conditions also increase the chances of an overall negative evaluation of online learning.

There is not strong evidence to link self-efficacy with evaluative perceptions of online learning. In support of the link is the positive evaluation of

Table 6.10. Relationship Between the Evaluative Perception of Online Learning and Self-Efficacious Beliefs

Evaluation	*Participants Describing Themselves as Self-Efficacious About Online Learning*	*Participants not Describing Themselves as Self-Efficacious About Online Learning*
Evaluated the experience of online learning positively ($n = 5$)	5	0
Evaluated the experience of online learning negatively ($n = 2$)	1	1

online learning presented by five of the six participants who described themselves as self-efficacious about online learning. However, among those who evaluated online learning negatively, Deborah described herself as self-efficacious about online learning, while Shannon was ambivalent.

Relationship Between the Evaluative Perception of Online Learning and Technological Proficiency and/or Regular Access to Human Supports

Is there a relationship between evaluative perceptions of online learning and the participants' technological proficiency and/or access to human supports? Table 6.11 presents a query of this potential relationship allowing us to ask whether online learners who are technologically proficient are more likely to evaluate their experience of online learning positively.

There is not strong evidence for a link between evaluative perception of online learning and technological proficiency (or lack thereof) of the learners. Two of the three participants who self-assessed as technologically proficient evaluated online learning positively. All three of the participants who self-assessed as not technologically proficient, but have regular access to human supports also evaluated online learning positively. The sole participant who did not have regular access to human supports and did not self-assess as technologically proficient evaluated online learning negatively. Perhaps a positive evaluation of online learning is possible when the learner is either technologically proficient or has regular access to human supports, but not in the absence of both of these conditions.

Table 6.11. Relationship Between the Evaluative Perception of Online Learning and Technological Proficiency and/or Regular Access to Human Supports

Evaluation	*Participants who Self-Assess as Technologically Proficient*	*Participants who Self-Assess as not Technologically Proficient, but Have Regular Access to Human Supports*	*Participants who Self-Assess as not Technologically Proficient, and do not Have Regular Access to Human Supports*
Evaluated the experience of online learning positively (n = 5)	2	3	0
Evaluated the experience of online learning negatively (n = 2)	1	0	1

Relationship Between the Evaluative Perception of Online Learning and Gender

The final explored relationship is that between evaluative perceptions of online learning and gender. Are males or females more likely to evaluate online learning positively, or is there no evident relationship between the factors? Table 6.12 charts the potential relationship.

There are no grounds for predicting a link between gender and evaluative perceptions of online learning. Only two of the seven research participants are male. Both evaluated online learning positively. Three of the five women also evaluated online learning positively. Perhaps, depending on factors unrelated to gender, men and women are equally likely to evaluate online learning positively.

Conclusion of Discussion Regarding Research Question One

What is it like to be a blind online learner? The seven online learners' depictions of the experience within interactive research interviews yielded nine categories. In alphabetical order, the nine categories are: (a) use of adaptive technologies, (b) experience of course accessibility, (c) course design including use of communication tools, (d) evaluative perceptions of the experience, (e) eye condition, (f) experience of interactivity, (g) nationality, (h) self-efficacious beliefs, and (i) self-assessed technological proficiency and/or regular access to human supports. Eleven potential relationships between these factors were then queried. The queried relationships were between: (a) use of adaptive technologies and experience of course accessibility, (b) experience of course accessibility and self-

Table 6.12. Relationship Between the Evaluative Perception of Online Learning and Gender

Evaluation	*Males*	*Females*
Evaluated the experience of online learning positively (n = 5)	2	3
Evaluated the experience of online learning negatively (n = 2)	0	2

assessed technological proficiency and/or regular access to human supports, (c) self-efficacious beliefs and self-assessed technological proficiency and/or regular access to human supports, (d) evaluative perceptions of the experience and experience of course accessibility, (e) evaluative perceptions of online learning and course design, (f) evaluative perceptions of online learning and eye condition, (g) evaluative perceptions of online learning and experience of interactivity, (h) evaluative perceptions of online learning and nationality, (i) evaluative perceptions of online learning and self-efficacious beliefs, (j) evaluative perceptions of online learning and self-assessed technological proficiency and/or regular access to human supports, and (k) evaluative perceptions of online learning and gender.

Analysis of the factors emerging from the conversations with seven blind online learners and the relationship between these factors paints the following picture of what it is like to be a blind online learner. It must be noted that this picture is sketched from the accounts of seven people. These seven people appear to be the first blind online learners asked to share their stories for research purposes. Their experiences, as interpreted within this analysis, reflect outwards to allow course designers and instructors, postsecondary administrators and prospective online learners insight into the lived experience of online learning. The story is not meant to be exhaustive, exclusive, or definitive. It constructs a depiction of online learning for these seven online learners at this time and place, and hopes to provide an indication of what online learning might be like for others.

Online learning is possible and potentially prodigious for blind adults. The majority of learners (who have no vision or low vision) retrospectively evaluated the experience positively. The strongest determinant of how the experience was evaluated was whether or not the online course design promoted interactivity. Most of the blind online learners were self-efficacious about the experience prior to beginning. Blind adults from both Canada and the United States of America participated in online learning. In order to effectively participate in online learning, these blind adults either had to be technologically proficient or had regular access to human supports. There appears to be a multidimensional relationship between self-assessment as not technologically proficient, not having regular access to human supports, not having self-efficacious beliefs about participating in online learning, and not succeeding in the course.

Blind online learners in this research accessed computer information and communications through adaptive technologies, the most common of which was JAWS screen-reading software. One of the learners who has low vision used ZoomText screen enlarging software. Three of the most common course components were experienced as accessible in that they were compatible with adaptive technologies. These accessible course components were digital content modules, e-mail, and e-mail coordinated through a LISTSERV. Printed texts were often inaccessible and resulted in time-delays for conversion to accessible formats. With respect to communication tools, some learners experienced bulletin boards as accessible and others did not. Adults with low vision were more likely to experience bulletin boards as accessible than adults with no vision, because most bulletin board interfaces use visual cues such as flags and colors for navigation. In addition, adults who self-assessed as technologically proficient were more likely to successfully navigate bulletin boards than those who self-assessed as not technologically proficient, probably due to the higher level of complexity of this communication tool as compared to e-mail communication. Synchronous text-based chat, synchronous voice-based chat, and simultaneous slideshow presentation and voice discussion tended to be inaccessible. The majority of contemporary courses as experienced by the informants facilitated interaction through one or more of these communication tools.

Research Question Two—Design Characteristics

This section of the chapter addresses the design of online courses and programs. It begins by positioning the courses and programs of the research participants along a continuum of interactivity. It then moves from the specificity of the seven research participants' experiences to extrapolating to design of online learning overall. The components of online learning that the participants perceived positively met the tips for online learning as composed by Coombs and Banks (2000). When experiences were unsatisfactory, one of these 16 tips had not been followed. The experiences of the seven blind online learners are therefore linked to these tips. The recommendations for design of online learning are not confined to considerations for blind learners exclusively. Instead, the intention of the design recommendations within this section of the chapter is to promote educational improvements for all learners.

The experiences of the participants in this research can be positioned along a continuum of interactivity. Interaction means that there is meaningful two-way communication between participants in the learning experience (Garrison & Anderson, 2003). For example, students dialogue together and debate critical ideas. The instructor and student negotiate and clarify learning objectives. The continuum is marked by four types or generations of distance education (Garrison & Anderson). The standard model of first generation is correspondence, or self-study whereby a textbook and lesson guide are mailed to each learner and she in turn mails-in her assignments. Some postsecondary institutions continue to practice first-generation distance education, using e-mail rather than post, and capturing materials on CD-ROM and DVD rather than text-books.

Two of the participants in this research were students of first generation online learning. Shannon enrolled in a Web-delivered cooking course. The course was self-study tutorial based. Shannon described a feeling of missing-out. She identified the missing elements of smells and tastes. In addition, Shannon described missing what authors such as Garrison and Anderson, 2003; Northrup, 2001; and Twigg, 2001 identified as the essential characteristic of online learning—interactivity. Shannon said,

> This is not for me. This is not useful for me to take a class … because I'm missing too many things. I'm missing the smells of the food. I'm missing. I'm isolated. I'm here in my house. It didn't seem like a very good way to learn that particular subject on the Internet through online.

Deborah enrolled in a first generation offering of an online course presenting the Americans with Disabilities Act (ADA) requirements—a thick volume of legislation. She described the experience as "pretty painful" due to lack of interactivity. "There was never any kind of face-to-face. Never any kind of teleconference. Anything that ever brought us together. It was strictly e-mail—strictly LISTSERV type interaction."

Second generation distance education broadcasts lessons from a central point to learners at a remote, or multiple remote locations (Garrison & Anderson, 2003). The broadcast is conducted through technologies such as television or videoconference. Third generation distance education fosters interaction through synchronous (same-time) and/or asynchronous (time independent) communication tools. Some theorists differentiate between third, fourth, and even fifth generation depending on the relative provision of three elements: "information retrieval of vast amounts of content; the interactive capacity of computer mediated communications and; the processing power of locally distributed processing" (Garrison & Anderson, p. 38). Fifth generation online learning is still a forecast rather than the current state of affairs and predicts learning portals and artificial intelligence.

Within the current research, there is little distinction in terms of interactivity after second generation. The distinction between the five students who experienced greater than second generation online learning can be made between those who experienced a "pure" online model, and those who experienced a blended model. Bernice has taken only one online course, but if she chooses to pursue the certificate of which this course is a part, she will study entirely online. Sarah has taken three courses toward a degree in which all of the courses are exclusively offered online. For Sarah, one of the most positive features of her online program is that there are no face-to-face courses. She enjoys the anonymity of studying online, particularly since she lives in a community of 6,000 people. She appreciates critical debate that is not interpreted through the lens of stigma. Martin's university is increasingly designing online counterparts to its face-to-face courses so that learners can choose their preferred mode of delivery. To date, Martin has completed three online courses, and will select online delivery whenever the option is available throughout his degree.

Madeline and Matthew experienced a blended model, whereby short concentrated-time study institutes were conducted face-to-face with the majority of courses online. Madeline and Matthew expounded the benefits of the blended model. Both Madeline and Matthew enjoyed beginning the program with a face-to-face study institute whereby the students got to know one another personally. Madeline's experience was that the collegiality carried through the online portion, thereby creating a safe zone for critical debate and shared problem solving. For Madeline, the main advantage of the online nature of the majority of the program was the convenience, not only as a personal asset, but in that the program ran because the online component ensured that enough learners were able to register. Matthew reflected on the pedagogical implications, stating that asynchronous discussion promoted higher level thinking and critical debate because it gave learners time to ponder and research prior to posting their responses.

All of the participants who experienced asynchronous communication echoed Matthew's appreciation of the time delay to review, revise, and reconsider. Garrison and Anderson (2003) believe that asynchronous text-based communication has advantages over face-to-face classroom discussion in terms of engagement in critical discourse and reflection. They described research demonstrating "because students have more time to reflect, to be more explicit and to order content and issues, teachers were able to ask higher-level written cognitive questions" (p. 26).

Coombs and Banks (2003) described 16 tips for the design and instruction of online learning. The direct experience of the seven online learners within this research support and exemplify these tips. The tips will be numbered to organize this presentation. However, the tips are not presented in the same order as that written by Coombs and Banks and neither are tips presented in any order of priority. The authorship of the tips requires elaboration because their personal and academic experience warrants their claims, and because two of the participants in this research completed their courses with Coombs and Banks as instructors. Dr. Norman Coombs and Dick Banks are the principal operators of Equal Access to Software and Information (EASI). EASI is located within the Rochester Institute of Technology. The organization offers online courses and maintains a Web site and an academic peer-reviewed journal intended to educate people about the intersection of disability and educational technology. Two inter-related grounding principles that have evolved through their work are that simplicity works more effectively than high-tech applications and that improvements to the design of online courses and Web site accessibility advantages those with and without disabilities. They are proponents of the metaphorical "electronic curb-cut." Just as portions of the sidewalk curb resting flush with the road promote ease of access for strollers, bicycles, and shopping carts as well as wheelchairs, design of Web sites with shorter download times benefit those who use adaptive technologies as well as those with low-band Internet connections, and intuitive interfaces benefit new technology users and people with learning disabilities.

Dr. Norman Coombs is totally blind and has been since he was 10 years old. He dedicated his career to academe as a history professor. He was initially resistant to digital educational technologies including e-mail, asking what a history professor needs with a computer. Upon experimenting with the technologies, the evidence for the pedagogical advantages was compelling. Two of his most engaging stories are one in which a deaf student with whom he (a blind professor) corresponded via e-mail commented that those correspondences were the first and only accessible scholarly exchanges she had experienced throughout her postsecondary education. The other story is in the transformation of discussion about African American history and issues which he knew to be an engaging topic, from dry, stifled face-to-face sessions to active, participatory online critical exchanges.

Dr. Norman Coombs met Dick Banks online through a LISTSERV and invited him to be the other principal of EASI. Dick is legally blind with low vision. He is technologically proficient enjoying the play with new tools. The partners live states away from one another and yet, through e-mail, correspond as if they have desks across the room.

Tip 1—Remember E-Mail

The first tip is to "remember e-mail." The wording of the tip implies that as online learning progresses, e-mail will be forgotten or replaced by more advanced communication tools with more complex functions such as bulletin boards and synchronous chat. Coombs and Banks (2000) wrote that e-mail should not be abandoned or outdated as it is "the best and most simple and most universal interactive tool on the Internet" (p. 3).

Five of the seven research participants experimented with various communication tools. While Martin and Matthew had positive experiences with bulletin boards, neither had success with synchronous chat. Sarah resorted to having her husband narrate the bulletin board postings and therefore could not participate independently, but had to wait until he was available. Madeline was relieved when after trying a bulletin board with the result of disgruntling the students her instructor reverted back to e-mail. Bernice did not use a bulletin board, but did not find functionality in either voice-based chat, or simultaneous voice discussion and slideshow presentation.

Some of the frustrations with advanced communication tools are unique to blind students in that the tool interfaces are incompatible with adaptive technologies such as JAWS screen reading software. Martin could log-in to the chat-room and the instructor could note his presence on the virtual role-call, but his screen reading software could not pick-up any content. Martin heard nothing once inside. Sarah's challenge was that read and unread messages on the bulletin board she used are differentiated only by color, and the distinction is thereby not picked-up by the screen reader. In addition, the entries do not read as discrete postings, but as an uninterrupted stream. She explained,

> We get to the conference board and my husband will read the unread messages. Now we've listened to JAWS read it through, but what happens is it will start at the top and then just keep going and going and going. I'm not sure what's read, what's not read, unless I remember from the day before.... I find that frustrating.

An emerging area of research within educational technology is the intricate relationship between usability and accessibility. Microsoft's new text titled *Accessible Technology in Today's Business* provides case studies to illustrate that when interfaces are intentionally rendered accessible for those with disabilities, they become usable for the general population (Moulton, Huyler, Hertz, & Levenson, 2002).

In the case of this research, the usability of communication tools provides an apt example of universal significance. Many of the participants' frustrations were not related to their blindness. Martin's frustration with synchronous text-based chat was amplified by his low vision, but not confined to users with a visual impairment. He commented on the frustration of the layout and pace of the text. Every time a user entered new text into the conversation, the rest of the text lines would jump up on the screen. Matthew could read three or four words of the line before it would move out of his line of vision. Sighted students also comment on the frustration of rapid reading while simultaneously trying to key in their own contributions. Often by the time a student has completed his entry and posted it, the conversation has moved on to a new topic. The conversation thus becomes disjointed and disorganized.

Madeline thought that she was the only student having trouble navigating the bulletin board and wondered whether it was a result of her blindness or her level of technological proficiency. She later discovered that the other seven students in the cohort were experiencing the same frustrations. The bulletin board was suspended and e-mail with a LISTSERV revived. The bulletin board interface is foreign to the experience of new users. Yet, most universities do not provide training in its use. Students are often challenged to determine how and where to post, and commonly forget or do not know how to designate a topic so that the discussion remains threaded. The other frustration inherent in bulletin board use is that the student must be online to retrieve and compose messages. If the server is down, or the Internet provider temporarily suspends service in the area, the student cannot access the bulletin board.

Bernice experienced frustrations with the synchronous voice-based chat. The students enter the conversation by holding down the "control" key on their own keyboard and then speaking. Bernice shared that she could hear the others speaking through her headphones, but had trouble figuring out when it was her turn to speak. Entering a live conversation can be challenging at the best of times, but when face-to-face it is easier to pick-up on subtle social cues and navigate one's way through participation. Conversations through a digital medium can be more challenging to manage whether the user is blind or sighted. It is likely that certain individuals monopolize the conversation and others never get a turn to speak.

There are numerous advantages to e-mail as the course communication tool. E-mail is largely accessible in that it is compatible with most adaptive technologies. It is easy to differentiate between read and unread messages visually and through screen reading software. Each message is clearly discrete and thereby does not run together as a stream of text or dialogue. It is easy to navigate and familiar to most computer users. It is easy to designate and recognize a subject line and the author, and maintain a thread of dialogue through using the "reply" feature. Dialogue can be forwarded to other users, including those who are not registered in the course. Expert opinion can therefore be sought to supplement class discussion. Students do not require a separate password or log-in interface to access course communications. It is easy and efficient to send a message to multiple people with a single command. Messages of a personal nature can be sent privately to a single user. Attachments including assignment submissions are easy to include. Users can request notification of receipt to verify that the message arrived. Archives are automatically created and easily accessed and printed. Users can organize and file their messages in a manner that works best for them personally. The layout, including font size and type, can be modified by the user. The print on the monitor stays still and in one place. Once e-mail is received in the inbox it is located on the user's hard-drive, and can thereby be accessed online. Outgoing messages can be composed and saved in the outbox to be sent when the online connection is restored. The asynchronous nature of e-mail provides time for learners to revise, rethink, and even research.

Tip 2—It's About People and Not Technology

None of the participants in this research enrolled in online learning exclusively because they were enamoured with the technology and wanted to play with online tools. If this was the case, then the content of the courses would not have mattered. Four of the participants (Madeline, Martin, Matthew, and Deborah) enrolled in order to learn the course content, and online was the only or the most expedient means of achieving that end. Sarah also saw online learning as a means of expanding her academic circle beyond her small community, and being able to keep her identity as visually impaired in her back pocket. Bernice is considering adding online courses to her own college program and sought the course as a model to emulate or modify. Shannon wanted to challenge herself, to see if she could overcome her frustrations with computer technologies.

In each case, the technology, at least at times, got in the way of the content. Sarah explained,

> I think that to me, a big problem with blind and visually impaired people working with an online course is that you interact more with the technology than with the content, or with the other students, or the instructor, or whatever. That your focus is on interaction with the technology. And that to me is the biggest frustration.

Sarah qualified her comments by classifying the problems as existing for "blind and visually impaired people." However, in the literature, the majority of students are encompassed when the concerns of technology as a barrier to learning are depicted. Within the literature depicting the student experience of online learning such as Dickie, 1999; Friesen, 2002;

Hara & Kling, 1999, 2000; and Robinson, 2000, three main grievances occur with the most frequency. First, students experience challenges in connecting to online courses and accessing and interacting with the content and communication tools therein. Second, interfaces are inexplicit, and communication is blocked. Third, students feel isolated, disembodied, and/or alien to a learning space and community. One of the most impacting images in Robinson's multimedia presentation of her research is of a flashlight beam circling a closed door and words scaling up in size over time, reading—"LET ME IN." Robinson presented the experience of students as a feeling of being shut-out by technology and thereby not "being in" the learning experience and having no "gathering place" conducive to learning.

Each of these concerns can be interpreted as symptomatic of failed interactivity. Northrup (2001) compared and combined models of interactivity in online learning to report four types of interaction: (a) student to student, (b) student to instructor, (c) student to content, and (d) student to management/feedback. When the term "interaction" is queried through Webopedia, an online dictionary of computer and Internet terminology, the passage addresses a fifth type of interaction—with the technology.

> Short for human-computer Interaction [HCI], a discipline concerned with the study, design, construction and implementation of human-centric interactive computer systems.... HCI is a very broad discipline that encompasses different specialties with different concerns regarding computer development: computer science is concerned with the application design and engineering of the human interfaces; ... psychology is concerned with the cognitive processes of humans and the behavior of users. (para. 1, 2)

The omission of student to technology interactivity within the online learning literature is problematic considering that: (a) the first two student grievances as listed above (access and connectivity, and inexplicit interfaces) almost exclusively fall into the domain of student to technology interaction; and (b) unless this type of interaction is addressed in course design, the third student concern (perceptions of unfulfilling learning experiences) is likely to continue.

It is the hope of most educators that the technology can one day "disappear" from the salient educational experiences of postsecondary online students. Negroponte (1995) wrote that the "secret to interface design" is to "make it go away" (p. 93). He continued, "ease of use has been such a compelling goal that we sometimes forget that many people don't want to use the machine at all. They want to get something done" (pp. 101-102). However, the interactions essential to reflection, critical thinking, and construction of understanding can only be achieved if student to technology interactivity is treated as an equal factor in the design and delivery of online courses.

Tip 3—Beware of Techies

Coombs and Banks' (2000) next tip is directly related to the previous. They advise course developers and instructors to "beware of techies." The warning applies to not over-using the technology. Do not include features that do not serve your teaching function. The authors use the oft-quoted statistic that "20 percent of the software commands are used 80 percent of the time, and 80 percent are used only 20 percent of the time" (p. 3).

Sarah's experience demonstrates that at times, inappropriate technological applications can be posed by the students as well as by the instructors. Sarah could not access the bulletin board postings without the assistance of her husband. She shared information about her visual impairment with the course instructor prior to the course start date, but disclosed to her student colleagues only when she felt her hand was pushed. Sarah was somewhat frustrated that the instructor did not intervene when one of the students took the course in technologically excessive directions. After Sarah spoke up, she learned that some of the students without sensory impairments shared her frustrations with the inappropriate acceleration of technology.

Tip 4—Make it a Team Project

While Coombs and Banks (2000) encourage instructors to take control of their course design so that they only include technological elements that suit their purposes, they advocate including the technical experts in the design team. They also advocate using students with disabilities at the design phase. While inexperience, negative experience, and/or fear of using computers can be problematic for all users, it can be particularly challenging for blind learners. The visual interface dominates computers, with little thought or attention to the auditory. Numerous software applications render the interface visually appealing. The screen is resplendent with color, graphic images, and even animation. There are hundreds of fonts, sizes, and textures. Bernice stated,

> they're always going to be coming up with things that are attractive visually and inaccessible and we have to try to talk to developers to make the virtual blackboards and things accessible in some way, or have an alternate way of communicating with people with disabilities.

What if you use your computer without a monitor? Do the navigation cues disappear? Is there any appeal to the auditory interface? Shannon described the frustrations of a tool designed by and for the sighted.

> It is frustrating because a computer is designed for people who can see anyway and so I have tasks I need to accomplish and I am trying to navigate. I am trying to learn, and then I am realizing that there is nothing.

Shannon uses JAWS screen reading software, so that when she referred to there being "nothing" she meant that the synthesized voice was silent, providing no cues as to what was on the monitor.

None of the learners within this research were asked to be on the design teams of the courses in which they enrolled, and to their knowledge there were no learners with disabilities (or likely learners at all) involved in the course design. Matthew's university is moving to a single learning moderation system to be used by most faculties and programs across the campus. This means that he will have to learn a new interface and how to manage compatibility with his ZoomText software. The courseware that Matthew will be using is Blackboard, which Martin experienced as having elements of inaccessibility. Matthew is seeking to influence the conversion of the courses from First Class to Blackboard at the beginning rather than waiting to deal with the inaccessibility resulting from not designing universally in the first place.

Tip 5—Keep it Simple

The next tip is—keep it simple. Four of the seven participants were enrolled in courses that were designed without the use of learning moderation systems. Learners' evaluations of courses designed in this way were just as positive as those enrolled in those using courseware, provided that the interfaces were intuitive and the process interactive. Madeline's course used Web sites and e-mail with a LISTSERV. Madeline commended the course design. Within the interview it was revealed that she had no idea what the term "learning moderation system" means or that courseware for online learning existed. Sarah's course used Web sites, e-mail and a WebBoard. She was pleased with the design of the Web sites, and her only frustration was with the bulletin board. Deborah's experience was unsatisfactory, but not because the course was designed prior to the popularity of courseware, but because it was not interactive. The enrolment interface was so complex for Shannon's desired online cooking course that she decided to suspend her involvement even prior to participating in the actual instruction.

Tip 6—Be Accessible

Within the online learning complex, simplicity is synonymous with another of Coombs and Banks' (2000) tips—accessibility. Norman Coombs (personal communication, March 19, 2003) explained his belief that accessibility is "where the rubber meets the road." Bernice queried whether her positive online learning experience is ubiquitous or whether it was unique and best attributed to the instructional source—Norman Coombs and Dick Banks and their University-based company—Equal Access to Software and Information.

> So it was for me, overall, a very positive experience, but as I say, it was meant to be accessible so from that perspective it was a good experience. I have heard about people with disabilities doing online courses having difficulty with PDF documents for example, ... and HTML pop-up menus that don't work with screen readers. You just can't access the buttons. Getting instructors to provide information in a text-format as well as whatever other format they're working with. A lot of instructors, I think, like to use a lot of bells and whistles and multimedia that add to their presentation, and some of those things can be problematic.

However, Madeline, Matthew, Martin, and Sarah also evaluated their online educational experiences positively, and they were each enrolled in online programs offered through four diverse universities. The key appears to be that the courses were for the most part accessible. Madeline equated accessibility with learning satisfaction and inaccessibility with isolation. She shared that the only time she felt isolated was when she experienced inaccessibility with the communication tool.

The practice of accessibility should not be conceptually limited to the disability context. Moulton, Huyler, Hertz, and Levenson (2002) wrote,

> Simply put, accessibility means providing access—making products and services available to, and usable by, everyone. Accessibility is about removing barriers. A more accessible environment benefits everyone—including people with disabilities and those without. All people benefit from an environment in which it is easier and safer to move and function. Ensuring accessibility is another way of accepting and encouraging diversity in our society. (p. 25)

O'Connor (2000) called online learners with disabilities "early adopters" implying that they are taking advantage of technology-infused education, and leading the way for other learners who are slower on the uptake. He predicted that this early adoption will move them from the fringes or "outer edge" to the "leading edge."

Tip 7—Design for Universal Access

Broad application of the concept of accessibility is conceptualized within the field of universal design. Universal design is "the design of products and environments to be usable by all people, to the greatest extent possible, without the need for adaptation or specialized design" (North Carolina State University, 1997, p. 1). It is highly recommended that a usable design be planned upfront. It is much more expensive with less chances of success to try to retrofit an online course or other educational technology such as a Web site, than to design it from the beginning so that it fits the needs of a diversity of learners. Universal design moves best practices in online learning beyond a disability issue to enhancing educational technology for all learners. Opitz (2002) provided numerous examples of how designing an online course such that it is accessible to students with disabilities benefits all learners.

> Images can be effective in providing alternative examples or explanations of content. The addition of an alternate text tag to the image enables a screen reader used by a visually disabled person to read the textual description to the learner, describing the attributes of the image. Adding a title representative of a description of an image also allows learners without disabilities a more detailed explanation of the image. Sounds can also be used, but captions or alternative text benefit the deaf and those with hearing by providing a written script to follow and to refer back to at a later date. Easy-to-read content benefits all learners by "chunking" the information into blocks of important information that can be easily read and understood by any audience. (p. 12)

Tip 8—Do Not Replicate the Classroom

For a time there were a series of studies that concluded that there was no significant difference between outcomes of face-to-face and online classrooms (TeleEducation, n.d.). Researchers since have pointed out the flaws in the majority of this research. However, authors such as Garrison and Anderson (2003) and Twigg (2001) believe that there still remains a lesson to be learned. Even though all of these authors advocate for online learning, they are not surprised that no significant difference emerged. They state that regardless of whether the courses were offered face-to-face or online, most maintained the same traditional teaching approaches—mainly featuring the lecture. The difference, and we might even say the advantage, of online learning comes in the potentialities of infused technologies (Jardine, Clifford, & Friesen, 2003). This leads Coombs and Banks (20000 to advise instructors not to replicate the classroom.

Only one of the participants within this research (Deborah) experienced an online replication of the classroom, and she was one of the two people for whom the experience of online learning was negative. There was no interaction. She described the course design as, "basically, it was take a professor and have them write out everything that they would say in a lecture," and then forward that lengthy lecture in text-form every 2 weeks via e-mail.

Madeline humorously described an example of how online learning technologies can be used to their best advantage.

> And we had great discussions on the LISTSERV about assignments and how we did things. And I remember one day starting a thread while we were taking our Independent Living Skills course. I remember one day going and making myself a slice of toast and peanut butter for breakfast. The normal thing that I'd do is get a spoonful of this out, put it on the toast, and spread it around evenly with my finger. But, I thought, oh man, I'd better not do this anymore. So I got out a knife and established a pattern to do it, and of course, I sent this message out to my LISTSERV and it started a whole conversation. I thought my instructor would really nail me for this, but I said that this is how I would teach a person to do this, but for all practicality, it's not the best way. Keep this is mind. So we did a lot of this kind of thing.

Madeline's anecdote provides insight into the nature of online course communication. First, her story refutes the notion that online courses are isolated, sterile environments. Her description of the nature of the conversation and the tone with which she shared the experience illustrates how a learning space can be cultured online. The conversation, which she described as a frequent occurrence, springboards from the course content to related applied scenarios. The communication was not confined to the assigned or the mandated. Further, the topic and the ensuing discussion are playful, fostering a connection between the learners.

Second, her comment that her "instructor would really nail me for this" depicts the course communication as explicit and public. One of the arguments for in-residence education is that the activities and conversations of learners can be monitored and checked when they diverge from philosophical foundations or demonstrate fallacious thinking. In other words, the professor serves as mentor, nurturing the development of the student. For example, this argument might be applied to Madeline's program in which the graduates will be teachers of blind children. The instructor needs to check and even "correct" the students when they suggest even seemingly innocuous activities that have the potential to erect barriers to a socially valued role in the community like spreading peanut butter with one's finger rather than with a knife. If this conversation were to occur on-campus the instructor would likely not hear the transgression and thus not have opportunity for teaching. This type of conversation, being a digression from the curriculum would likely occur on the class break or in the hallways between classrooms. When the students do not have a venue for side-bar conversations, the dialogue occurs online, where the instructor can monitor and mentor.

Tip 9—Modularize

Coombs and Banks (2000) recommend modularization. Organize the content into manageable modules and follow-up each with assignments promoting interaction. Madeline provided an example of how this was applied in one of her courses.

> And each of the twelve lessons of the Independent Living Skills—each one would be on a different aspect of Independent Living. It would say Lesson One, Lesson Two, Lesson Three, Lesson Four. Each would be on a separate link, and you could go to whichever one. And each would have a description of what you were going to learn, and the readings, and at the bottom of that would be the assignment.

Madeline, Sarah, and Deborah's courses were designed such that each module was accessed through a separate URL, print unit and/or e-mail attachment. This was an effective component of the course design, except in the case of Deborah's course in which the module was not followed-up with interaction. Matthew, Martin, and Bernice's courses were designed such that they entered the course through one Web site and then accessed each module through a discrete icon.

Tip 10—Be a Virtual Host

The next tip, which Coombs and Banks (2000), themselves provide examples to emulate is—be a virtual host. Welcome your learners and invite them to interact. Norman Coombs (personal communication, March 19, 2003) described himself as a little bit academically stuffy, and a little bit informal and casual. So, he coined his username—Prof. Norm Coombs. He maintains the Professor title, but makes it more approachable shortening it to Prof and inserting his first name. Bernice, having completed a course with Dr. Coombs, described him as playing an active role in the initial course discussions and then gradually pulling back as his learners demonstrate levels of active engagement. She described the resultant social atmosphere.

> I loved it. I thought it was great fun and I enjoyed interacting with the people. I guess you get out of it what you put into it and that is really important too. I think that if you are kind of really not very outgoing and very hesitant to express your views then perhaps it might be more difficult. But then one of the things that Norman Coombs said was that sometimes in an online format people who are very shy in class because they are afraid of the way people will look at them are not shy in the online situation because they don't have those nonverbal interactions so it makes them more comfortable and they participate more effectively.

Just as Bernice frequently referred to her course instructor, Prof. Norm Coombs, throughout the interview, Madeline referred to her course instructor, Dr. Cay Holbrook. Both refer to the professors with respect and admiration. Both professors had an obvious online presence that cultured a community of learners within their courses. Although Matthew did not refer to his instructors by name, he described the active morality of two of his instructors, one of whom is a minister whose theological background and social services perspective are evident in his teaching, and the other who has a long history of teaching in grade school.

Tip 11—Set Boundaries

Whether instructors such as those that Matthew, Madeline, and Bernice described as invested in the relationship and interested in the character development of their learners and the social action deriving from their teaching followed Coombs and Banks' (2000) next tip, "set boundaries," was not explicitly mentioned in the interviews. This was the only tip that was not directly supported within the interview transcripts. However, neither was it refuted. The research interviews were with the online learners about their learning. Perhaps the practice of instructors who set effective boundaries such as balancing how much time they spend communicating with their students and how much time they reserve for their own personal lives apart from teaching are not salient for the learners. In other words, the nonemergence of instructor boundaries within the interviews might be an indication that these boundaries were so effectively managed that they went unnoticed.

Tip 12—Provide Redundant Communication Modes

The next tip is to provide redundant communication modes. Mayer (2001) explained that multimedia "refers to the presentation of material using both words and pictures" (p. 1). He described his rationale for research into multimedia. "The case for multimedia rests in the premise that learners can better understand an explanation when it is presented in words and pictures than when it is presented in words alone" (p. 1). The other case for multimedia is built on accessibility. Both learners with disabilities and learners with diverse learning styles and preferences benefit with planned redundancy of communication modes, or in other words, when equivalent information is presented through both auditory and visual modes.

None of the interviewees described provision of planned redundancy within their courses. They were able to access the information in auditory form, only because they had screen reading software installed on their computers. Each of the participants who use screen reading software replied that it would be a pleasure to listen to an auditory presentation made by a human voice rather than through the synthesized voice of their software. However, Deborah pointed out that if it was a matter of replacing one synthesized voice with another, then she might as well use her JAWS screen reading software because she already knows the interface and has the speed set at a personally comfortable rate. Bernice speculated on what redundant communication would be most advantageous.

> If they use presentations, you know text articles, it's important that if they're available in a PDF format that they also make them available in text format. It's a little easier than a PDF document. PDF documents aren't all that easy to read, even though screen readers will now read them. It's more convenient when it's converted to text. If they have a presentation that's really visual, then it's important for them to have another, separate link that describes it in text, rather than the person just not being able to get anything out of it at all. The assumption is that a lot of multimedia is accessible just because it's on the Web. That isn't usually the case. A lot of times the buttons and graphics are not labelled appropriately, and they're just not—the person is simply not able to access them without some assistance. Sometimes if, for example, someone who is sighted can click on a button and all of a sudden the rest of the presentation is available, but if you can't get to it in the first place then it becomes very difficult to get the material. It's frustrating. Audio presentations using real audio are very helpful. Then again, if you're looking at deaf people taking courses then there needs to be an alternate text presentation. And that's a fair bit of work because someone has to listen to the audio and type it out and make a text version of it. But if you really want to do it right, it's a very good thing to do.

In summary, Bernice advocates for redundant communication in terms of alternate presentations in text for all audio presentations. She stated that real audio would be preferred but that it is not a necessity. It is, however, a necessity that all text presentations are either fully compatible with screen reading software, or that an equivalent version is provided.

Tips 13 and 14—Understand the Problems of Students With Disabilities and Have a System to Deal With Special Problems

The next tip is to understand the problems of students with disabilities. The counterpart tip is to have a system to deal with these problems. The system should be established and enacted long before the course start-date. The problem most referenced by the interview participants concerned access to texts and other resources. Students with disabilities often require reading lists and materials in advance so that accessible formats can be arranged. Martin explained,

> I get the books through Recordings for the Blind and Dyslexic for the most part. Sometimes our library in Des Moines—at the department for the blind—will tape the books if we can get them to them on time. That's always a big thing, because sometimes you don't get your book list until way too late for any taping to be done.

Madeline, Martin, and Sarah each shared instances of receiving print materials too late in order to have them translated into an accessible format in time for the course start date. Matthew does not need the materials translated as he accesses it through use of ZoomText software and by using a handheld magnifier. Bernice's and Deborah's instructors provided the materials digitally so that they were compatible with their screen reading software.

Madeline described her frustrations regarding inaccessible texts and what happens when books are not available in advance. She described receiving a required text-book in an accessible format over half-way into the course. She mentioned two names in this excerpt. Cay is her professor. Kevin is a pseudonym for her husband. Both are sighted.

> But I finally got the *Foundations of Education* on disc, but it took about two months. And it took a long time before it was done. I found that really odd. I think that all these books are on computer, because I think that they have to do them up on computers before they are printed, but firms are very reluctant to give these away. And I mean I've said, "It's a book. I'll buy it at the same price." But I finally got it through the American Federation of the Blind. But it took me ages. Now, what I finally did, before that, was Cay lent me her copy of the print book, and thank goodness I was working online because I was able to scan it. And it's not as good as having it on disc because if it's scanned you are going to get errors and it takes a lot more time. And it's just generally more difficult. Sometimes I'd ask Kevin to scan the chapters in for me, that I needed, because he can do it so fast just looking at it. And also I was a little reluctant in case I bent a page or anything like that. But if I hadn't had access to my computer all day to scan these

> files, if I'd have had to try to get all this stuff read, go to class and do the work, I don't think I could have done it because my materials would have been in print. But at least, at least online I could do what I needed to, to get access to the materials. But once I figured out the system, it was okay. But it threw me when I was all ready to get into these courses and I didn't have a book. That was freaky. It was a real wake-up call.

The solution that worked most effectively for the learners was the provision of materials in an accessible format such as a digital medium that is compatible with screen reading software. If the materials cannot be provided in digital formats, then the second best solution was to plan ahead and provide the materials at least two months prior to the start date of the course so that the students could have the texts translated into their preferred accessible format such as Braille, digitized or audiotape.

Tip 15—Understand Adaptive Technologies

As well as recognition of the potential problems of students with disabilities and planning solutions to be enacted by the postsecondary institution, it is also important to be familiar with some of the solutions applied by the students themselves. Deborah explained that even when redundant communication modes are implemented, adaptive technologies are often still necessary. Deborah was asked whether she would prefer to listen to a recorded narrator through an audiolink than to listen to the synthesized voice of her screen reading software.

> Absolutely! Absolutely! Every time that that is a real viable—and when I say viable I mean that it still has to provide you the functionality. So, you still need to work with JAWS, because it's still going to be JAWS that gives you the information about where you are on the screen, which section you're in, which question you need to answer.... But we can't be confused about the fact that having that sort of audible information does not necessarily give you the information you need to navigate the site like JAWS would do.

An analogy regarding accessible buildings might serve to clarify. The inside of the room might be completely accessible to someone in a wheelchair. The room is constructed on a single level, and all shelves are mounted at a level that someone in a wheelchair could access the contents. Unless, however, the doorway is built wide enough to let the wheelchair pass, the person cannot enter the accessible room. Each of the learners used a metaphorical digital doorway to enter. Madeline, Martin, Sarah, Bernice, Deborah, and Shannon use JAWS screen reading software. Matthew uses ZoomText screen enlarger software.

In chapter 5, Madeline's story provided an estimate of the costs of adaptive technologies. She believes that she has approximately $25,000 worth of hardware and software in order to study online. Shannon is concerned for people who do not have the financial resources.

> I guess one of the things I get concerned about is, as we head more into technology, is the technology going to be technology the people in the community can actually get their hands on. Because the computer equipment for people who are blind—it is not cheap to have JAWS or to have a Braille display. To make it usable costs money. To me that contributes to another layer of isolation in that we have this technology and people will say we will have forms online and we will have this. I always say, "but what about people that don't have access to this?"

Tip 16—Be Interactive

The final tip brings us full circle to the essence of online learning—interactivity. Coombs and Banks (2000) stressed the importance of being interactive. Five of the seven learners experienced interactivity within their courses, and overall these learners evaluated their courses and programs positively. Martin shared his experience in this regard.

> I've always had good interaction. The instructors are always very cooperative, and they answer questions when you e-mail them. And students a lot of times will respond, if I've ... made a response to a student's comment or something. I've always enjoyed good interaction with students and teachers alike.

Conclusion of Discussion Regarding Research Question Two —Course Design

In summary, Coombs and Banks (2000) provided 16 tips for online learning. Fifteen of the 16 tips emerged as themes in the transcripts of the interviews with seven blind online learners. The one tip that did not emerge was for the instructor to set boundaries. This tip was not refuted, but did not emerge in the participants' accounts of what it is like to be online learners.

Of the 15 tips validated by the seven learners in this research, the first discussed tip was to remember e-mail. The learners supported e-mail as the most consistently accessible, usable, interactive communication tool.

The second tip is that it is about people and not technology. The participants enrolled in order to learn about the course content and not because of a technological imperative.

The third related tip is to beware of techies. Instructors should not let those whom Boshier and Mun Onn (2000) refer to as techno-utopians convince them to add online course components that are technologically intriguing but are not necessary within the particular course. One of the common features that emerged among course components positively evaluated by the informants was their simplicity.

Tip 4 is to make it a team project. If the course designers want to ensure that the course is accessible, then students with various types of disabilities should be involved in the planning process. None of the seven learners were invited to inform the design of their courses, although they would have participated if invited and will volunteer suggestions for future courses.

Tip 5 is to keep it simple. Sometimes the most effective and efficient tools are the simplest. Once again, e-mail emerged as an example within this research. Professors and students in faculties beyond computer science should feel invited to participate through the adoption of plain technologies.

Tip 6 is to be accessible. One of the keys to accessibility is to ensure that the materials are compatible with adaptive technologies. Although not all of the course components were experienced by the learners as accessible, they were each able to access at least one content module format and one communication tool.

Tip 7 is to design for universal access. The metaphor of electronic curb-cuts holds that if access is improved for students with disabilities, then usability is improved for all learners. None of the courses experienced by the research participants were universally designed. They were each required to use adaptive technologies in order to access the courses.

Tip 8 is do not replicate the classroom. Online learning has its own pedagogical practices that are being discovered as more and more online programs and courses are developed. As evidenced by Deborah's experience, the dispensary model of education is ineffective online.

Tip 9 is to modularize. Each unit of content should be presented discretely and followed-up by interaction and an assignment. The informants commended this feature of their courses. Most experienced the content modules as discretely presented either through a Web site design that included separate links for each unit, or through time-released units.

Tip 10 is to be a virtual host. As demonstrated by Bernice's instructors —Coombs and Banks (2000), instructors must make extra efforts to create an online presence. As a result, interaction is demonstrated and fostered between students.

Tip 11 is to provide redundant communication modes. Presenting equivalent content in auditory and visual modes benefits learners with sensory impairments and people with diverse learning styles and preferences. Information was not duplicated in audio and visual formats within the courses experienced by the research informants. Many of the learners explicitly advocated for multimedia developments in online learning.

Tip 12 and 13 are to understand the problems of students with disabilities and to have a system to deal with special problems. The biggest problem experienced by learners within this research was inaccessible print textbooks. The first solution was to provide the text in an alternate format in a timely manner. The second solution was to get the text to the student well in advance of the course so that the students could get the text translated.

Tip 14 is to understand adaptive technologies. Most of the participants in this research used JAWS screen reading software.

The final tip is to be interactive. The majority of learners participating in this research experienced online interactivity. They linked their positive perceptions of their courses and programs to this interactivity.

Research Question Three—Impact

The third question guiding the inquiry queries the impact of blind adults studying online. Of the three guiding research questions, thematic content of the transcripts addressing impact emerged in the smallest proportion. Three areas of impact emerged from the conversations with seven blind online learners. The first object of the impact is the fellow learner in terms of attitudes and actions. The second object includes all learners as the participation of blind learners in online courses appears to impact course design. The third object of the impact is the student herself, who not only learns the curriculum-based course content, but may also develop her computer proficiency.

Two of the participants cited specific instances in which their presence in the courses made a difference to the attitudes and the resultant social actions of student colleagues. Matthew commented generally about the ambassadorial benefits of his presence in a community of learners and then described the impact on one student in particular.

> I think there's a real impact upon your co-learners, on your cohort. And I think there's a real impact that goes well beyond that, that you don't even perceive. There are a lot of people who pick up information from, I don't want to say me, but from a person with a visual impairment, who might go home afterward to their family and say, "You know, I haven't thought of a visually impaired person being able to do this."

Matthew's reference is to the presence and visibility of blind people in socially valued roles. It not only impacts the attitudes of the student colleagues with whom Matthew has direct contact, but has a spreading effect on more generalized public attitudes and beliefs about what blind people can and cannot do. Matthew described one student colleague in particular who considered Matthew in application of the course content, and frequently e-mailed him with reflective questions. In one e-mail, the student colleague wrote, "I'm glad you're in the course. Because it gives people a different perspective. People have to think a little more creatively, and start saying, 'Yes, we are thinking of the whole spectrum of people within society.' "

Sarah enjoys the anonymity that online learning provides, particularly as she lives in a community of 6,000 people where privacy is rare. In chapter 5, her story of correspondence growing to friendship with two student colleagues is shared. In this instance, Sarah felt forced to reveal her identity as visually impaired. She now sees that there are some positive impacts of such self-disclosure. Since meeting Sarah online, issues of accessibility have compelled one of the women to social action. Sarah described her as "actually contacting" their postsecondary institution "to find out what policies they have and what policies they would like to have in the future." She has also tested their Web site with several validation tools and contacted them with the results.

A blind learner's experience of inaccessibility might also impact the usability of the interface for all students. Madeline's unsatisfactory experience with the bulletin board communication tool precipitated re-evaluation on the part of the instructor as to whether the tool should be maintained. Madeline was one of eight learners. Even if she, as one student, could not participate then that is still a significant portion of the class. The instructor opted to return to e-mail as the communication tool. The entire class breathed a sigh of relief, as what was not accessible for Madeline, was not usable by them either.

The third area of impact is in the area of transferable skills. A few of the participants briefly commented that their computer skills and confidence had increased through the experience of online learning. Madeline commented on feeling terrified upon her first experience of using the World Wide Web, juxtaposed against her current comfort level. Bernice said, "your computer skills would definitely improve" and "your confidence perhaps might increase in terms of whether you were comfortable interacting."

Bernice represented the pervasive attitude of the seven participants when asked whether she felt that her technological skills had developed in the process of taking an online course. She replied, "I haven't really thought about that too much." Throughout the conversations, the participants were united in their perspective on the place of technology. They appear to be in agreement with Negroponte (1995) that the technology should disappear from salience within the experience. At this stage in the development of online learning, a great deal of experimentation with technologies makes this nonpedagogical element salient. In addition, much of the interface remains new and foreign to the students, meaning that they have to devote time and attention to the educational technologies rather than the education itself. In other words, while the participants agree that enhanced computer skills are natural fallouts of online learning, they wish to de-emphasize this topic, as they wish the focus to remain on the learning of course content. Computer-mediation is a means and not an end.

Two additional themes in the domain of impact emerged through the literature and were introduced to the research participants for their perspectives. There was a great deal of divergence in opinion between the informants regarding segregated education and ambassadorial roles. Will online learning become the new model of segregated education? Will the public perception of blind people be deleteriously affected if blind scholars study online rather than on campuses? A danger, always a threat when considering schooling for persons with disabilities, is that the systems will become segregated and the options further restricted. Professors may no longer see the need for universal design and to make reasonable accommodations for blind post-secondary students in traditional face-to-face classes if they see the place of such students outside the building in front of their computers in their own homes. A paper published in *The Ragged Edge Online* titled, "Distance Education: Boon or Bane?" reads,

> Worries that distance learning will become a way to enforce separate and unequal are not unfounded. "If they can take classes over the Web, we don't have to make classrooms accessible," we can imagine administrators thinking. Online learning may offer a new means of segregating difficult students. What better way to show students that they are special than to deport them to the Cyber-classroom where they can't be disruptive. (Blaser, 2001, p. 5)

In preparation for the seven interviews, telephone conversations were held with two computer access specialists who were enrolled in an online program and had each completed several online courses. One of the men is blind and the other has low vision. In terms of demonstrating capability, Smith (personal communication, October 29, 2002) is not certain that online learning is the avenue. He explained, "with all the prejudice there is in the world, if I am to stay home all the time, participating in online learning from home, then I can't go out and prove that I am a human being just like anyone else."

Most of the research participants in this research became impassioned with these issues. There was dialectical tension within and between transcripts. Rereading the words after the transcripts were chopped into thematic pieces and pasted together according to relevance to the issues of impact rather than unified transcripts of the conversation with each separate respondent is reminiscent of listening to a debate between people brought together in a face-to-face context. Some of the comments indicate agreement that online learning may become a new segregated model of education and/or that public perceptions of blindness will be disadvantaged. Sometimes the same respondents who argued affirmatively with these issues also presented counter-arguments. Snippets of dialogue from the interviews with the seven participants are included here. The authorship of the quotations is not indicated as doing so would unnecessarily distract from the dialectical tension.

> Perhaps even though you're an online learner, as compared to people who are in the classroom face-to-face, prior to having that technology, you might not have been involved whatsoever.

> We generally don't encourage people to take online classes as it were. The only time we would is if that's all that's available, obviously. But, one of the reasons we don't encourage people to do that, is we do want people to get out into the community and we do want them to be able to move around and be amongst the public and so forth.

> I think that's certainly something [the segregation of blind learners to online classes] that's been considered from some sources. I don't think there's a great danger of that happening. I think there's still way too many people who are blind ... who are still going to be attending classroom settings.

> Every blind and visually impaired person is out there as an advocate or an ambassador for the blind, whether they want to be or not. They're out there. For every hundred people, let's say there's one blind person. And that blind person, to the hundred people, that's what blindness is all about. They look at that one person. They don't look at all the other people who they don't see, or they don't know..... There might be a desire to go into that classroom and be that representative.

> Quite honestly, I don't think I've ever heard anything more ridiculous! [the debate about blind learners as ambassadors] I keep thinking, what is the point of a course? Is the point of a course to show your own competence or the point of a course to be learning something new?

> I think that certainly an important part of post-secondary education is the social interaction, and attending school and meeting those other people

and interacting with them and learning. I learned a lot of important life lessons outside the classroom but on the campus of a university.

It's a potential danger [segregation of blind learners to online classes], but I guess part of what might prevent that, is that no matter how much people like me talk about ways to make it accessible, it just isn't very accessible in many instances right now. So it's not gonna happen.

With me as a full-time worker, it's almost a must to be online.

In summary, some of the lines of dialogue support the ideas of Blaser (2001) in *The Ragged Edge Online* and Smith (personal communication, October 29, 2002) that enrollment in online learning and support for online learning as an option for people with disabilities should be critically evaluated for one or both of two reasons. First, it may become a new type of segregated education. Second, people who are studying online are not in the public eye demonstrating capability. Another counter-online argument that was entered by some of the participants is that online learning may be used as an escape, or in other words, a means of succumbing to anxieties and self-doubt thereby erecting a safety net and withdrawing from campus orientation and public contact.

Other segments of the conversation support online learning. Some of the participants feel that these issues are moot points for various combinations of the following objections. First, blind people do not need to carry a torch for normality. Second, people enroll in postsecondary institutions in order to earn an education, not for an audience for social justice. There are other venues for ambassadorial roles. Third, there is little danger in online learning becoming the main option for blind students because despite its promise, it continues to be largely inaccessible. In other words, there will still be plenty of blind learners in the classroom. Fourth and finally, in a blended model the learners experience both face-to-face and online courses, thus fulfilling the ambassadorial role while benefiting from the convenience of delivery.

An argument that did not explicitly emerge directly related to segregation within the seven interviews is that blind learners are demonstrating their competence online through interactive discussions, perhaps to an even greater extent than in the face-to-face classroom. Matthew shared the story of a student colleague who was impressed with Matthew's contribution and thankful that he is in the course. This is an example of fulfilling an ambassadorial role online. Boman (2002) argued that face-to-face appearances distract from introspection and listening to the insights of others. Garrison and Anderson (2003) espoused the virtues of text-based communication, supporting online learning as fostering critical thinking and scholarly debate. The blind online learner thus has an even stronger avenue for demonstration of capability than in the face-to-face classroom. Batron (personal communication, October 29, 2002) expressed his view that the increasing prevalence of online courses will not decrease opportunities for blind learner participation in the traditional classroom. In fact, he believes that the opposite will transpire. He explained,

> If instructors and professors look at what can be accomplished in the online courses, they would be more aware that blind students can be capable of any level as a sighted student, and be more willing to accept them in their face-to-face classroom.

For many of the research participants, the bottom line is the pragmatics of online learning. Perhaps it is the best option for some because it is convenient. Those who are geographically isolated or constrained by other commitments such as work or family cannot manage an on-campus education, whereas they can participate online.

Conclusion of Discussion Regarding Research Question Three—Impact

Kim-Rupnow, Dowrick, and Burke (2001) posed the question, "do the increase in distance education programs and use of advanced technology indicate better access and better outcomes in higher education for persons with disabilities?" (p. 25). This question queries the impact of online learning on persons with disabilities. While Kim-Rupnow et al.'s literature review led them to be optimistic regarding the impact of online learning on persons with disabilities, the response was inconclusive. There was very little research addressing this question, and almost none of it was research based. The research depicted in this text posed impact as one of the guiding questions. Of the seven research participants, four had either completed or were in the course of completing a postsecondary program of studies leading to either an undergraduate or graduate degree. These informants unanimously said that if the programs were offered face-to-face rather than online they would not have opted to enroll in the programs. Two of the participants learned content online that they otherwise would not have been able to access. Both applied this content to improving their career functioning. Not only did online learning impact course and program access, but the digital technologies of online learning positively impacted access to information and communication within these courses. All of the participants found electronic documents more accessible than printed text and e-mail more expedient than post. Only one of the seven participants was not impacted positively through online learning, and even she would consider online courses in the future. In other words, for six of the seven informants in this research, online learning improved access to postsecondary education for blind adults thus promoting positive outcomes. This is an affirmative answer to Kim-Rupnow et al.'s previously unanswered question.

Impact as operationally defined by access and outcomes in postsecondary education is only one component of impact overall. Three other types of impact emerged in the interviews with the informants. The participation of a blind student in online learning was reported to positively impact the attitudes and actions of student colleagues. Instructors made accessibility improvements to the online courses, which positively impacted usability for all of the learners. The blind adults not only learned the content of the course, but also became more technologically proficient.

This section of the chapter also addressed a value-based debate in the provision of online learning for blind adults. It was queried whether there would be deleterious impacts of online learning. Two questions were posed: (a) will online learning become a form of segregated post-secondary education for blind adults, and (b) will the participation in online learning and thus absence from face-to-face classrooms withdraw accomplished blind adults from the public eye, thus negatively impacting public attitudes. The research informants presented arguments on both sides of these issues. Even those research participants who acknowledged potential negative impacts chose to enrol in online learning. Within the informal cost-benefit analysis, the convenience of online learning appeared to be weighted higher than any other factor. Regardless of whether online learning was judged as segregating, and regardless of whether the informants felt that they could be better ambassadors if participating in face-to-face classrooms, in most cases online learning was the only means in which they could participate in post-secondary education, and they appreciated having that option.

Conclusion of Chapter 6

As an interpretation of the content of interactive interviews with seven blind online learners, three research questions structured the chapter. A depiction was constructed of what it is like to be a blind online learner. A response to this question encompasses an evaluation and a description of the experience. For the seven participants in this research, online learning was more often than not a positive experience. Practical application is inherent in the response to the second question regarding what elements of course design promote best practices in online learning. The accounts of the informants resonate with sixteen pragmatic tips emerging out of the literature. The key to the design of online learning appears to be simplicity. Clearly organized content modules and usable communication technologies such as e-mail were unanimously preferred by the research participants. The third question concerns the impact of blind adults studying online. Impact of online learning in general is anybody's guess at this point. This research indicates that online learning might improve access to postsecondary education for blind learners. The research participants provided a few situated examples of impact they have noted as a result of their participation in the courses such as on the attitudes and actions of student colleagues and on improvements to the course design. Finally, the intersection of blindness and online learning pose unique questions regarding impact, querying segregated education and public image.

This chapter presented the second stage of reflexive analysis, applying the three guiding research questions to the stories of the seven blind online learners as presented in chapter 5. The transcripts were examined to inform: (a) what it is like to be a blind online learner, (b) what design characteristics are best practices in online learning, and (c) what impact is yielded through blind adults participating in online learning. The next two chapters apply qualitative concepts of reflexivity. The accounts of the informants are not simply reproductions of their experiences as online learners. The salient experiences of the learners and what they choose to tell through interviews are informed by what it is like to be a blind adult and what technology means at this time in history within American and Canadian culture. Chapter 7 presents an analysis of the stories of the seven learners from a critical theoretical perspective. This chapter applies constructionist notions of blindness and technology to the experiences of the participants. Chapter 8 presents an analysis of the discourse. The words used to compose the stories inform an interpretation of the experience.

CHAPTER 7

BLINDNESS RESEARCH THROUGH CRITICAL THEORY

INTRODUCTION

Chapters 5 and 6 described stages one and two of the reflexive analysis of interviews with blind online learners. The focus was on the empirical material. Chapter 5 presented the stories of seven blind adults who have studied online. Chapter 6 presented an interpretation of these stories by identifying themes or categories of the experience and conducting a comparison within and between stories considering the themes in relationship. Empirical research in the domain of online learning, particularly as experienced by blind students, is important in that it constructs a phenomenology, thus informing, or facilitating an empathetic view among those who are outside the experience such as prospective students, instructors, course designers, and administrators. Such insight has the potential to influence policies and practices.

While empirical research into blind online learners is necessary, it is not sufficient. Alvesson and Sköldberg (2000) described "three powerful reasons for not regarding empirical material as the whole truth, or as a decisive path to knowledge" (p. 134). The first reason is that "different phenomena should be elucidated in light of the totality-subjectivity com-

Seeing Beyond Blindness, 147–161

bination, which means that only limited aspects of a phenomenon lend themselves to being illuminated in a particular study" (p. 134). For example, reflection regarding who the seven research informants are, also requires asking who they are not. Whose input is missing from the analysis?

The second caution concerning empirical research is that "the social conditions, ideologies and communicative processes [are] operating behind the back of the subjects, in their subconscious, and which mean that the results of interviews and questionnaires are ambiguous" (p. 134). The current research is contextualized by public beliefs about blindness. As described in chapters 1 through 3, public mindsets about blindness permeate the perceptions of all, including those who are blind. These beliefs and attitudes affect the planning and delivery of educational programs.

"A third reason for avoiding over-confidence in empirical data is that studies of what is deemed to presently *exist* fix our attention on the actual and draw it away from what *can be*" (p. 134). This research depicting the experiences of blind online learners is not motiveless, or in other words, the intent moves beyond "pure" knowledge building to social action. The goal of this research is emancipatory and pedagogical. By exploring the experiences of seven blind online learners specifically, the hope is to disseminate knowledge regarding how to improve educational practices for blind adults more generally. In addition, the serendipitous goal emerging from the stories is the application of the pragmatic findings such as design characteristics to improve online learning conditions for all students, not restricted to those who are blind. Yet, there is a matrix of blockages to the emergence of an image or direction for the future, not the least of which is the technological imperative of Middle American culture determining the stories we tell ourselves and others.

The goal of this chapter is to trouble the empirical data as shared through the constructed stories of the informants and as interpreted through theme analysis. The intent of this chapter is to raise questions. Alvesson and Sköldberg (2000) wrote,

> One of the aims of critical theory is to increase our awareness of the political nature of social phenomena and to develop the ability of researchers to reflect critically upon those taken-for-granted realities which they are examining and of which they are also—as members of society—an inevitable part. (p. 111)

The researcher cannot escape, or step-outside, mindsets of the age or shared cultural subconscious understandings, any more than can the informants. Alvesson and Sköldberg wrote, "a problem is that research often unconsciously purveys and reinforces existing patterns. Researchers are themselves prisoners of their own society and its taken-for-granted concepts, thus helping to reproduce the status quo" (p. 129). This being said, it is the researcher's obligation to scrutinize the way in which the empirical data are invited, featured, highlighted, and storied, and to try to identify taken-for-granted assumptions. A literary parallel is to try to be like Jane Austen (1775-1817), the English novelist who had the ability to see the irony in her contemporary society and to convey this in her writing. The reader is invited into the dig for "deep structure" or in other words, "those unquestioned beliefs and values upon which the taken-for-granted surface structure rests" (Alvesson & Sköldberg, p. 136).

This chapter is organized into three sections by the challenges to empirical research as described above. The first section asks what and who within the domain of blind online learning was selected for study. The second section revisits underlying assumptions about blindness as presented in chapters 1 through 3 in relation to the processes and outcomes of this research project. The third section troubles responses and interpretations that are boarded-up preventing a view of what online learning could mean for blind students and for learners in general.

The Informants

The intention of this research was to create a forum for the discussion of what online learning might mean to blind adults. What it is like to be a blind online learner appears not to have been written previously. These stories were therefore not accessible to prospective students, course designers, instructors, and administrators. The goal of this research is to facilitate access to these stories.

The experiences of seven people are not intended to represent every blind person's experience of online learning. The results are not generalizable in the quantitative sense. The term "sample" is not often used within the domain of qualitative research, because its derivation from quantitative research carries assumptions of being able to establish within a reasonable doubt that the subset of data collected can be used to generalize findings to the wider population. Yet, the term "sample" is illuminating within qualitative research. The empirical data is shaped on a series of decisions. In order to write the research proposal, decisions were made to have face-to-face conversations with people, to have the conversations with adults, and only with the learners themselves, and to talk with people who had some experience of online learning.

In keeping with these decisions there were seven research participants. Five participants are totally blind and two have low vision. Five participants are women and two are men. Four participants are Canadians and three are Americans. All of the participants enrolled in mainstream courses as opposed to courses particularly targeting prospective students with disabilities. One participant enrolled in a course outside of a postsecondary institution. Two participants each enrolled in a single course offered through a private organization based out of a postsecondary institution. One participant is an undergraduate. Three are in the process of completing or have completed a graduate level program.

The research decisions excluded. Critical theoretical research encourages conversation with minority groups, such as the blind online learner. This research intends to give voice to those who have not yet been heard. However, broadcasting the voice of some shuts out the voices of others. For example, chapter 5 presents the approaches of Dr. Cay Holbrook and the supports of a spouse from Madeline's perspective. The professor and husband are not invited to tell their own stories. A few disappointed and one disgruntled e-mail were received from willing informants who would have liked to participate in the research, but could not because the research budget did not allow anymore travel for face-to-face conversation. Restricting the conversations to adults meant that blind children and adolescents could not inform the stories of online learning and contribute to a future image. This exclusion is unfortunate as children's and adolescent's perspectives on education are shaped by knowing no other world than that infused with computer technologies, as opposed to the interviewed adults who experienced schooling that did not involve computers and who adopted computer technologies later in life.

One of the most restrictive decisions was to include only people who had experienced online learning. Five of the seven informants presented positive depictions of their online learning experiences. One of the two informants who had a negative experience was nevertheless positive about online learning generally and will likely enroll in future online courses. Convenience emerged as the key motivating factor for online learning. In other words, this research contributes to the maintenance of a social order in which: (a) postsecondary education is constructed as important; (b) the goal of education is professional development, meaning that mature adults are expected to balance multiple roles such as career, family and education; and (c) infused computer technologies are welcomed.

This excludes those for whom escalating costs of postsecondary and private industry continuing education preclude their enrollment. It excludes those who do not have access to computers or perhaps interest in using them. It excludes blind people who do not know about adaptive technologies and/or have no means of securing and learning how to use them. It means that those who do meet university entrance examinations or are positioned in a socioeconomic status that is less likely to promote education do not have the privilege of constructing the stories of Middle American pedagogy. Blind people who have been maintained in the role of client and cared-for in human services have limited access to opportunities for emancipatory knowledge building. This research does not give them the opportunity for reinventing themselves or restorying their lives.

From a critical theoretical perspective, who are the seven informants in this research? Who received knowledge of this research? Who felt compelled to volunteer? Who was accepted? All seven adults have a minimum of a bachelor's degree completed or in progress. All are independent, competent, accomplished adults. Most have spouses and/or children. They are mature, established people. They are well-spoken, intelligent, and reflective. Each has a career in social justice. They are working toward amelioration of societal conditions for minority groups. They are all White, English speaking, apparently middle-class citizens of the United States or Canada. They all own their own computers and have access to the Internet. They all own adaptive technology software. Four learned of the research via e-mail and three via association with a professional conference.

Who does this exclude? Who does not get to contribute to the authorship of this first story about blind online learners? The sample does not include people who: (a) have no postsecondary education; (b) are dependent adults in care; (c) are alone and isolated; (d) are in their 20s or are of retirement age; (e) are language or computer illiterate or have trouble verbally communicating; (f) are not willingly unemployed or are substantially underemployed; (g) have no knowledge of or investment in social issues; (h) are members of racial, language, socioeconomic minority groups; (i) are below the poverty line; and (j) have no access to online communications or no experience of professional conferences. It is intuitive that the stories would be substantially different if the participants were among those excluded. While the results of this research with the seven informants would recommend the promotion of online learning for blind adults, interviews with people with any number of the above characteristics, might, for example, have yielded recommendations that online learning not be pursued.

Underlying Assumptions About Blindness

One of the research informants—Bernice—promoted a critical theoretical stance on blindness issues across every stage of the research production. Within her personal story, in her follow-up e-mails and in her validation of the written text, she troubled assumptions underlying the depiction of the organized blind, professional organizations, and the resultant beliefs about blindness. Ferguson (2001) traced the challenge to the dominant social order within the domain of blindness in the United States of America fronted by the National Federation of the Blind. Ferguson's book served as inspiration for this research. Reading the text shaped the research questions and the research decisions. The research proposal was submitted to Ferguson for approval. This research was funded by The Louisiana Center for the Blind and the Professional Development and Research Association on Blindness at Louisiana Tech University. At that time, Ferguson was their director of research. The philosophy and practices of both organizations are consistent with that of the National Federation of the Blind.

The benefit of this grounding is that the research is steeped in a critical perspective. That critical perspective is shaped by Ferguson's (2001) interpretation of Foucault's writings and his application of policy archaeology. It also embraces the challenging voice of the organized blind to counter the dominant voice of the professional blindness agencies such as the American Foundation for the Blind. The danger is that in recognition of incorporation of a single critical stance, the research might too easily lose its metacritical perspective ceasing to rotate the lenses through which the research is critiqued. The critical theoretical perspective of the research is indebted to the informant who asked questions and raised awareness primarily through juxtaposing American and Canadian systems of blindness.

As described above, all of the informants in this research are professionally involved in amelioration of social conditions for minority groups including the blind. This involvement means that their perspective is informed by direct experience of cultural practices and privileged to "insider" knowledge. Three of the informants live and work in the United States of America. Four live and work in Canada. The story of blindness systems in the United States is recorded in chapter 4 primarily through reviewing Ferguson's (2001) *We Know Who We Are: A History of the Blind in Challenging Educational and Socially Constructed Policies*. An equivalent volume presenting and critiquing the Canadian matrix of blindness was not located and is thereby not represented within the literature review.

This research would be remiss in not juxtaposing the matrix of blindness in the United States with the story of the Canadian blind. The identity of the blind within the two countries is distinct. For example, in 2005 a blind consumer group was initiated in Calgary, Alberta, Canada. One of the first discussions was whether the membership wanted to be a Canadian division of the U.S. National Federation of the Blind (NFB). It was decided that due to the discrepancy between the Canadian and the U.S. experience of blindness, this group of organized blind would not fit comfortably under the construction of the NFB. They initiated their own identity, called the *Alliance for Equality of Blind Canadians* (AEBC).

A source of the Canadian construction of blindness is Dr. Hartin, the Executive Director of the Canadian National Institute for the Blind Ontario Division. Hartin was invited to present to the World Blind Union general assembly (2000) on the topic, "Is it time to start thinking unitary: Consumers and service providers—a vital partnership" (p. 1). Hartin was invited as a representative of the Canadian blindness system as organizers felt that the Canadian model achieved what others were seeking to emulate. The goal of Hartin's presentation was in part to clarify the history, the strengths and the continued challenges to the Canadian system of blindness. As presented in chapter 4, with regard to the system in the United States, the Canadian blindness system also struggles with tension between consumer groups and professionals. Some disability studies activists such as Heshusius (2003) caution that this tension should not be resolved (i.e., a bridge is undesirable) as compromise would wipeout the critical perspective that the consumers "offer" to the professionals. Hartin presented that others feel that the adversarial relationship is counterproductive, misdirecting energy away from the shifts in public attitudes and social practices that requires unified efforts.

Hartin (2000) described "two dominant players" in the history of the Canadian system of blindness (p. 2). The Canadian National Institute for the Blind (CNIB) was founded in 1918 by blind war veterans. Many of the founders of the CNIB were themselves blind, and it continues to be staffed and directed by a large percentage of those who are blind. It is mandated that the President and CEO of the CNIB be a blind person. Just as the 1940s were important foundational years for the consumer movement in the United States with the establishment of such groups as the National Federation of the Blind, consumerism was also seeking a foothold in Canada. The Canadian Council of the Blind (CCB) was officially established in 1944. The CNIB helped to establish this consumer group.

The relationship between the two groups has been troubling since the inception of the CCB (Hartin, 2000). With the support of the CNIB (including funding), the CCB maintained its strength. However, some say that it did not have the distance from CNIB in order to challenge and present, where needed, a strong opposing voice. An example would be if the CNIB were to establish a service that the consumers perceived as perpetuating the custodial model. To use the colloquial, to challenge practices of the CNIB would be "cutting off the nose of the CCB to spite its face." In the late 1980s and the early 1990s, it was mutually decided that the CNIB and the CCB should become distinct entities. The implication was that the funding arrangement be discontinued. The result was that the CCB lost its foothold. "Unfortunately, the CCB was unable to maintain its strong national presence without the direct funding support"

(Hartin, p. 4). The CNIB continues to be publicly regarded as the voice for and of the blind. The challenge to this authority is not vocal. As testament, the Canadian Council of the Blind would not have been included within the pages of this research if its existence had not been pointed out by Bernice.

What are the implications of the commonalities and discrepancies of the Canadian and American blindness systems to the current research? It is the premise of this research that the stories of the informants are shaped by the shared understanding of phenomena as constructed by a given culture through history and as interpreted contemporaneously. This is not to say that members of a culture hold a unitary perspective. As illustrative, three diverse positions on the continuum of affiliation with the organized blind as shared by the participants in this research are quoted here. The sources of these position statements are not individually named due to the research participants' contract work with many of the blindness organizations.

> I've been affiliated with the National Federation of the Blind back in the sixties and seventies and since. And one of the reasons is because I like the philosophy of blindness that the National Federation of the Blind espouses, which is basically that blindness really isn't a catastrophe. It's more a nuisance than anything else. It's just a part of you. It's a characteristic, I guess. It's who I am. I guess I like that philosophy and also that a blind person with proper training and opportunity can do the average job in the average place of business as well as their sighted neighbour, or better sometimes.

> I feel like I have a stronger *individual* voice within the American Council of the Blind. I feel that I can show up at any national board meeting at the American Council of the Blind [ACB], and that not only will I be heard, but I will be listened to. And that I'm not being shoved in any particular mould of, "This is *the* approach to blindness." And because I don't think that there is one single approach to be dealing with blindness. I think it is individualist. It is up to people to make it individual, and ACB allows for that scope within its membership.

> It's been my experience that many of the consumer groups, by no means all, but many, have had a chip on the shoulder, a "You owe me!" attitude that I find quite offensive. So for the most part, I have chosen not to become involved in something like that.

The first two statements were voiced by citizens of the United States of America. The latter was voiced by a Canadian. Is this coincidence or substantive? Nationality is used as an interpretive category within chapter 6. Americanism and Canadianism in the context of blindness appear to shape, or at least inform, the counterarguments of the citizens. (It is telling that the U.S. based spell-check provides a red underline denoting a spelling error for "Canadianism" and not for "Americanism." Is there no such thing [for Canadians] in the minds of Canadians, Americans, or both?) While there are discrepancies in the individual interpretation and application of what it means to be blind, there are commonalities in language and shared insider understanding of social justice, of advocacy, and of tensions between professionals and the organized blind.

There are implications of the context of blindness on the interpretation of the response to the three questions guiding this inquiry. What it is like to be a blind online learner is informed by an interpretation of what it is like to be blind. If blindness is just a characteristic, then the phenomenon of online learning is minimally informed by the adjective. If blindness is predominantly an issue of social justice, then accessibility is a serious and litigious issue. The second research question, concerning course design, also rests on cultural meanings of blindness. If blind people are considered to be regular people who happen not to be able to see, then being able to access the material is important, while no special accommodation is desired or welcomed. If society is perceived as unjust owing remediation, then the institution and instructor should bend-over-backwards to ensure that the educational experience is a good one for the blind student. The third research question queries the impact of blind people studying online. The debates of chapter 6 regarding segregated education and ambassadorial roles are grounded in the social construction of blindness. Some of the participants were irritated by the asking of these questions because they feel that blind identity is not the issue. Online learning is about education, not about blindness. Others think blindness is a pivotal factor in debates concerning the morality of educational technology.

Technology Blockers

This third and final section of the chapter queries the extent to which the status quo blocks creative *vision*. In other words, can we imagine what online learning can be beyond the perception of what currently exists? The first level of the critique is pragmatic. Each of the participants experienced only one program of studies through a single institution. In other words, each person's perspective on what online learning is, was informed by their single experience. Questions regarding what the future might hold, or in other words, how they would like online learning to be designed, fell relatively flat. Creative dreams were stifled by the present experience.

The second level of the analysis concerns social structures and their unconscious foundations. Society does not have to be structured by levels of education, and by campuses, teachers and students. The computer does not have to be designed into every gadget, office, and vehicle. Yet, this is the world structure we know and take for granted. It is challenging to shift our thinking outside the structures and imagine a different manifestation of everyday living.

One of the critical theoretical perspectives on online learning considers this manifestation of educational technology to be a direct result of a technological imperative. In short, are computers embraced in education because they enhance learning, or because we feel compelled to their presence? Beyond the tangible, explicit objects of computers, some theorists such as Franklin (1999) question the linear, managerial means by which we carry out our every day lives. Alvesson and Sköldberg (2000) described the role of critical theory in the application decisions of educational technology.

> Yet it is also, and above all in a high-tech society, concerned with critically scrutinizing the pervasive influence of techno-rational subsystems and the technical cognitive interest, as well as with counteracting the tendency of technocracy to supplant political and ethical positions as a governing principle in society. (p. 125)

This research's declaration of online learning as topic, and then propositions concerning how to make the practice most effective, is in part, maintaining the social order. We need to continually challenge and reawaken the sleeping giant question of whether we want to go there. Can we unblock ourselves from the shackles of the present excitement of educational technologies, in order to ask whether or not we should pursue online learning?

Postman (2003) is critical of the adoption and proliferation of online learning within postsecondary campuses. He is the Chair of the Department of Culture and Communications at New York University and author of 20 books including *The End of Education* (1995). His chapter in *The Wired Tower: Perspectives on the Impact of the Internet on Higher Education* (Pittinsky, 2003) "addresses six key questions about technology and media, answers to which might provide some insights into the ways e-learning may intrude itself into our institutions of education" (p. 184). His image of online learning as a wilful intruder pervades the discourse of his chapter. The following section of this chapter addressed these six questions within the context of disability studies, and specifically the participants in this research.

Question One: Is There a Problem?

Postman's (2003) first question is, "what problem gets solved by this new technology?" (p. 187). He provided examples of "technologies that are not solutions to any problem that a normal person would regard as significant" (p. 188) such as satellite technologies facilitating an almost infinite number of television channels. Within the present context, we need to ask what problem gets solved by offering online learning to blind post-secondary students. It is an issue of social justice that blind postsecondary students should have full and open access to the full range of educational experiences available to any other post-secondary student. So the first response to this question is to broaden the scope and ask what problem gets solved by offering online learning to any postsecondary student. The demographics of postsecondary institutions are shifting. Citing 18 studies, Thompson (1998) profiled the distance learner as: (a) older, (b) female, (c) employed full-time, and (d) married. Levine (2003) added that distance learners are usually part time students. Online learning has the potential to meet the needs of this student population, whereas traditional post-secondary education may be impractical for the majority of contemporary students.

The profile of the participants in this research resonated with the profile of online learners as presented in the literature. Notably these demographic characteristics have nothing to do with the participants being blind. All seven participants are mature students. Five of the seven are female. Five of the seven are students while employed full-time, meaning that they are part-time students. Five of the seven participants have spouses, and six of the seven have grown children. Six of the seven participants commented that if the courses were not delivered online, their participation would not have been feasible.

While the demographic characteristics of the learners are not confined to blind students, one of the current problems specific to blind learners in face-to-face education is that information, including but not restricted to course texts, is inaccessible, untimely, and/or in an inefficient format (Chandler, Hu, Arndt, White, & Smith, 2002). Three of the four research participants whose course delivery included printed texts experienced this medium as inaccessible. Digital information via computer-mediated education, on the other hand, is accessible through bits thus capacitating choice in format and "user-pulling" rather than "provider-pushing" (Negroponte, 1995). All six of the participants whose course delivery included digital content modules, e-mail and LISTSERVS experienced these media as accessible.

Question Two: Whose Problem?

Postman (2003) submitted that most technologies solve some kind of problem for somebody. However, the problem is often one significant for the powerful, and not for the majority. Postman explained, "we need to be very careful in determining who will benefit from a technology and who will pay for it" (p. 189). Two problems were described above: (a) models of education provision that do not meet the needs of older, working, part-time students, and; (b) inaccessibility of information to blind students. Both are problems for the students, who are often the underdogs within the educational system. However, the problem appears to have been hijacked, or even harsher—bastardized—by the corporate culture of universities. In his introduction to Greg Cappelli's (Senior Equity Analyst for Credit Suisse First Boston) chapter in *The Wired Tower* (2003), Pittinsky (2003) wrote, "as much as many of us would like to hold on to the idealistic notion of a university operating outside the daily financial grind of revenues, expenses, and budgets, today's institutions of higher education are complex businesses" (p. 41). Cappelli specified two university goals in offering online learning: (a) to better serve their existing or potential student bodies, and (b) to penetrate a wider potential student base (p. 59). It is clearly the latter that pervades the discourse of the chapter. Cappelli dedicated a number of pages to privatization and the competition and collaboration between for-profit and public institutions and companies. He wrote, "postsecondary education is clearly an area where select e-learning for-profit companies can capitalize on the increased demand for lifelong learning" (p. 50). A solution that apparently solves the problems of two groups—one powerful, and one weak, may proclaim the motives of the latter group in public discourse, while using the motives of the first group to shape the plans. Six of the seven participants in this research experienced inaccessible components of their courses. None of the participants were consulted in the planning stages of online course development and delivery to ensure that the postsecondary course offerings met the needs of their blind students.

Question Three: Creating New Problems?

In *We Know Who We Are*, Ferguson (2001) empirically demonstrated the impact and the oppression of socially constructed notions of disability, professionalism, and vision on people with disabilities, those who care about them, and society as a whole. In one chapter, he traced the decline of Braille teaching and usage to an increase in prevalence of blindness beyond the capacity of school boards to provide special education teachers proficient in Braille, and a misapplication of the concept of stigma. Oppressive attitudes toward the blind created a myth that reading a Braille book, thus establishing oneself as identifiably blind, is more stigmatizing than functional illiteracy. Ferguson used an example of a child who was denied Braille instruction because she could read 10 words-per-minute using a text magnifier; a good Braille reader can read 250 words-per-minute. Ferguson's is a prime example of what Postman (2003) meant when he stated that the solutions to problems usually result in some new problems. The solution to the problem of stigma was to cease teaching Braille thus promoting functional illiteracy. Online learning as a solution for the problem of inaccessible information might further exacerbate this problem. This may become another excuse not to teach Braille. Educational administrators may take the position that blind students do not need Braille with technological devices to assist their education. Five of the seven participants in this research expressed concerns about the decline of Braille literacy, and each emphasized that digital technologies are not a replacement for Braille.

Question Four: Potential Harm?

Chapter 6 presented perspectives on the impact of online learning for blind adults. Several of the research participants recognized the potential for online learning to become a segregated form of education for blind adults. It may not be incumbent upon face-to-face professors to make their classrooms accessible if the place of blind learners is seen to be online. While two of the research participants expressed that they would advocate against online learning should they ever detect that online learning became the only postsecondary delivery option for blind learners, they doubted that such advocacy would ever be necessary because the inaccessibility of computer mediation means that many blind learners will continue to choose face-to-face delivery. While the participants considered the possibility of segregation to be an intriguing issue, its impact was perceived to be secondary to the convenience of online learning. Their decision to enroll in online learning was pragmatic. It was possible for them, as mature adults with multiple life responsibilities, to complete courses through online delivery. The provision of education where it would be otherwise impossible was perceived to outweigh any potential harm.

Question Five: Language Changes?

Postman (2003) implored the reader to explore the way in which incorporation of new media changes the language we use, and the reflexive shifts in shared meanings of phenomena. One cannot help but feel optimistic given the current context of the overlay of disability and technology. Wolfensberger (1972) dedicated a career to helping people understand socially valued roles, and how to use socially valued means to help devalued and oppressed people to assume these roles. Disability falls near the bottom of the totem pole in terms of what is socially valued in our culture. Technology, with its associated science and economy, sits near the top. Fostering technological roles with the blind cannot help but have a positive effect on language and then on social value. Each of the seven participants in this research commented on the personal benefits of improving their own technological proficiency. For five of the seven participants, improving the technological proficiency of other adults who are blind or have other disabilities comprises a large component of their career responsibilities. Three of the research participants explicitly commented on the positive impact of technology training on the social status of blind adults.

Question Six: Power Differential?

Postman (2003) highlighted the importance of this sixth and final question, "what sort of people and institutions acquire special economic and political power because of technological change?" (p. 197). There are widespread concerns of a digital divide, and further, of whole cultures and countries wielding dangerous power through information. Spender (1995) wrote, "instead of drawing upon the diverse resources and perspectives of the global village, the odds are that the views of the most powerful will be imposed on the rest of the world" (p. 140). Shannon expressed her concerns about many factions of society being left behind because they cannot afford the costs of technological solutions.

This question pulls together themes of the preceding five. Access to the full range of educational delivery options and to information in a functional format has the potential to protect the power of blind learners. The resulting changes in language and in discourse have the potential to promote socially valued roles. However, the user- or student-based plans might be usurped by systems and procedures that capitalize on the economic benefit for the provider, thus increasing the power of the University. Specific casualties of this derailment might be the segregation of blind learners to online systems and de-emphasis on Braille teaching in favour of technological solutions.

Conclusion Of Chapter 7

A critical theoretical research stance was taken within this chapter to trouble the topic of the inquiry and the means by which it was conducted. Three cautions regarding empirical research were considered: (a) what and who were included within the research, and wherein were the exclusions, (b) how do beliefs about blindness (constructed in part by American and Canadian blindness systems and structures) inform the voices of the informants and the subsequent interpretation, and (c) how does "what is" block a vision of "what can be," informed in part by a technological imperative. Postman's (2003) six critical questions were considered to inform debates about whether online learning should be promoted for blind adults. Postman's six questions as applied to this research are: (a) what problem gets solved by blind adults participating in online learning; (b) whose problem is it; (c) what new problems are created after solving an old problem; (d) who and what might be harmed by the proliferation of online learning; (e) what discursive changes might result from the adoption of online learning for blind students; and (f) what is the predicted effect of online learning on power differentials. While the participants in this research contemplated the risks of online learning for blind adults, overall they expressed their perception that the impact of online learning is more positive than negative. The convenience of online learning makes post-secondary course completion possible for mature students and many of the digital technologies make the course information accessible.

CHAPTER 8

DISCOURSE ANALYSIS

INTRODUCTION

Chapter 5 presented the stories of seven online learners who are blind. Chapter 6 interpreted those stories through identification of themes and comparison within and between stories. Chapter 7 adopted a critical perspective to probe the impact of the informants and the cultural meanings of blindness and technology on the research outcomes. In this stage of analysis, the stories of the seven online learners as told within face-to-face interactive interviews and through subsequent e-mail correspondence are revisited with a focus on discourse. While this is the stage of analysis presented fourth by Alvesson and Sköldberg (2000) and is thereby presented as the fourth analytic chapter within this research, discourse precedes the stories and makes their telling possible and meaningful, and it pervades the research and necessitates interpretation throughout. In other words, just as stage theory in such psychological domains as child development and grieving is misinformed when it is applied in a rigorous, sequential, step-by-step chronology, discourse analysis is not neatly stacked up on top of critical theory, nor is it an afterthought to interpretation.

As used in this research, discourse means words in and of relationship (Mills, 1997). It includes the meanings or conceptions of reality,

Seeing Beyond Blindness, 163–173

often held as truths or unexamined assumptions shared and communicated by a group of people. It recognizes language as both reflecting and constructing phenomena in our lived experience (Alvesson & Sköldberg, 2000). As such, when we put words to an experience, or in other words, story our lives, those words recall the events, the circumstances and sometimes our feelings about the happenings, and at the same time, the story creates the experience, or gives it meaning, positioning it within our phenomenology as humans. We know it to be true because we have storied it.

This chapter applies the lens of discourse analysis to the research on seven blind online learners. The first section explores the relationship between the researcher and the participants. While the methods of inquiry were such that attempts were made to facilitate the unraveling of each story as the participants wanted it told, the event of conversation between two people makes an element of cocreation germane to the inquiry (Alvesson & Sköldberg, 2000). In addition, this text was authored by the researcher; while the stories were offered back for validation and the content troubled throughout, the interpretations were written and disseminated through the privilege of the author. In addition, the time spent on validation by the participants was of necessity limited. The participants selected for this research are busy adults with multiple roles such as students, employees, parents, and social justice advocates. The implication is that once trust is established, they are likely to leave the authoring primarily in the hands of the researcher. Thus, it is important to examine that relationship between the researcher and the participants. Can trust be assumed? How invested were the participants in sharing their stories, and why would they be compelled to tell the "truth?"

The second focus on discourse turns back once again to the initial face-to-face interview transcripts. Two chunks of discourse were analyzed. The first is autobiographical. Each participant was asked to share whatever he or she liked regarding his or her personal story. Both the content and the order of this sharing are relevant. One of the contemporary issues that matters within the field of disability studies is steeped in the complexity of discourse. Some advocates hold that person-first language should be used without exception. In other words, the research is about seven online learners who are blind, and not about seven blind online learners. The rationale for person-first language is that blindness is only one aspect of the person, just as hair color, career, and nationality are also components. It is thus espoused that the order of the language should reflect this order of relevance. Other advocates hold that identity is extraordinarily determined by disability. Unless disabled identity is declared and embraced, personhood is smothered and efforts for social justice truncated (Shapiro,

1993). Black Americans and feminists made inroads to equality only upon declaration as collective groups. The National Federation of the Blind is intentionally neither *for the blind*, nor *of people who are blind*. So how did the participants within this research present themselves? Where are their descriptions of themselves as blind positioned within their stories? Is there a discrepancy between the Americans and the Canadians within the research?

The second chunk of analyzed discourse is the response to the question—"what is it like to be a blind online learner?" Once again, both how the research participants responded and the order in which their responses emerged are informative. Which descriptors within the question were most salient in the responses of which participants? In other words, did they answer the question with respect to blindness, with respect to online learning, or with respect to the interaction between blindness and online learning? Were their responses evaluative or description without judgment?

Did they highlight technology, course content or a combination? One of the most intriguing reflections in a hermeneutic phenomenological research study of mainstream online learners by Robinson (2000) was that when asked a phenomenological question, the content of their studies did not emerge in the responses of the students. Jardine, Clifford, and Friesen (2003) wrote of content as the third leg of the stool with teaching and learning comprising the other two legs. To extend the metaphor, the construction of education as depicted within Robinson's research was hobbled. The third leg was not referenced. Was the topic of study also missing in the depictions of the learners within this research, or was content salient in their responses?

The portions of the interview transcripts that comprised responses to the questions—what is it like to be a blind online learner, and who are you —were punctuated in sentence form in order to allow an indication of discursive response. In other words, counting sentences allowed a rough indication of extent and ordering of focus on a particular topic. As spoken language is more informal and less definitively punctuated as written language, criteria for what counts as a sentence were established. Within this analysis, a sentence is five or more words and is separated by an extended pause in speaking. It must be recognized that the division of sentences is arbitrary and an indication of number of sentences should be interpreted as reflecting an estimate and not an exact number. The sentence was selected as the unit of measure rather than centimetres of words on a page or number of words, as some speakers are more verbose than others, and some use more "filler" words than others.

Relationship Between the Researcher and the Informants

The topic of the inquiry is such that relating experiences of blindness and of educational achievement are personal and involve risk in trusting the researcher with the stories. Trust was established through the adoption of ethnographic research approaches (Emerson, Fretz, & Shaw, 1995; Fetterman, 1998; Spradley, 1979). The current research did not incorporate the ethnographic practice of long-term naturalistic observation and intensive social membership because the seven respondents were not all members of the same bounded community, but were each single members of seven educational communities, and four of the accounts were retrospective. However, two ethnographic practices were adopted. Connection was established through the researchers' acquisition of insider knowledge, while distance from the experiential particularities created the space for comprehensive telling. The researcher was informed about the domain of online learning and of blindness through: (a) prior experience as an online course designer and instructor, and (b) sponsorship by the Professional Development and Research Institute on Blindness and the Louisiana Center for the Blind. At the same time, the researcher was uninitiated into the particularities of the informants' courses, programs, and experience of blindness. As described below in the research situation of Robinson (2000) membership in the community into which she was inquiring might have led the informants not to share information which they felt she already knew.

The second ethnographic practice was to form a relationship with the participants. In most cases, numerous e-mails preceded the face-to-face interview. In addition to logistics of the interview, journal papers, links, thoughts, and ideas were shared. Correspondence regarding familial and other personal matters as well as scholarly considerations continued beyond the face-to-face interview increasing the likelihood of the participants' continued interest in validating and supplementing the research interpretations. Several of the correspondences have evolved into collegial relationships and one into friendship that will in all likelihood be lifelong.

All of the informants were willing participants in the research. Deborah admitted initial hesitation because of a busy schedule and prior unfavorable experience as a research participant. However, she assessed the topic of inquiry as important, and agreed to participate. Immediately following the interview, Deborah expressed that she greatly enjoyed the conversation and looked forward to the research results.

All of the participants recognized the research questions as important, potentially yielding practical consequences for the education of blind adults. All seven participants work toward social justice with and for individuals with disabilities and are thus invested in participating in educational improvement.

Autobiographical Depiction

Each of the learners was asked to share his or her life story. This question was asked only after the interviewer had a sense that a strong rapport and level of trust had been achieved. This question was inserted approximately one-quarter to one-half way through each interview. Participants were asked a variation of the question, "Maybe we could back up a little bit, and you could tell me more about you. Your story. Whatever you'd like to share, right back as far as you'd like to go." If respondents asked for clarification or queried what was specifically desired as a response, the following examples were offered, "work, family, education, blindness, interests." It is important to note that while blindness was not provided as the only categorical prompt, it was offered. The implication of prompting with the category of blindness and titling the research "Blind Online Learners" means that blindness as a topic of conversation did not emerge through free association on the part of the respondent.

Four of the informants opened their response to the request to share their personal story by describing their eye condition. Two of these four individuals (the two with low vision rather than total blindness) had extensively described their eye conditions early in the interview prior to being asked to share their stories. Notably, the four individuals who opened with their eye condition are the Canadians in the research, and the three who did not are the Americans. Two of the Americans opened by describing their work and the third by describing her personality attributes. While analysis of the responses of seven individuals (with factors representing nationality at the size of four and three) cannot be taken too conclusively, a hypothesis can be posed. It is possible that the perspective of the Americans has been shaped by the culture of blindness in which the vocal message of the collective organized blind is that blind people are normal human beings who happen not to be able to see, and that blindness is only one characteristic of the person (Ferguson, 2001). This message is pervasive even for those who are not official members of the organized blind groups. There is not, and never has been, a strong contingent of the Canadian organized blind (Hartin, 2000), thereby making the message of normality less predominant in the views of the participants.

In terms of what component of the personal story was mentioned second, three individuals described their families, two individuals their current employment or employment histories, one individual her current and past homes, and one her personality characteristics. Other elements in the personal description included perspective on disability (by three individuals), membership with the organized blind (by two individuals), and volunteer work (by one individual). In other words, the depictions were varied and there were no notable distinctions between the personal stories of the participants in this research and what might be expected from sighted informants.

Phenomenological Presentation of Blind Online Learning

After establishing familiarity and rapport through small-talk, and creating a framework for the research agreement by discussing issues such as consent and dissemination, each interview was opened with the question, "What is it like to be a blind online learner." With respect to which components of the question emerged as a salient topic early within the responses, blindness was prevalent. One respondent opened by describing his eye condition. Four respondents opened with another topic and then addressed their eye condition. Of these five respondents who addressed blindness first or second, three spoke of accessibility with regard to their eye condition, one addressed vision change and one mentioned blindness as an incidental autobiographical detail, as he is employed in a blindness organization, and his motivation for taking online courses is full-time employment.

The two respondents who did not address blindness first or second within their responses were Deborah and Shannon. Deborah mentioned blindness in her 25th sentence, and Shannon in her 54th sentence. Notably, what marks Deborah and Shannon as distinct from the other five is that they were the only two who had unsatisfactory experiences in online learning. The reasons for the unsatisfactory experience differed. Deborah's course was noninteractive. Shannon was a new computer user who did not have technological training nor support. The extent to which these experiences were unsatisfactory was held in common.

So how did they open their responses? Deborah dedicated her first and second sentence to a description of the content and her third and following sentences to the manner in which the course was delivered. Shannon dedicated her first sentence to the combined response of content and the process of attempting to enroll in the course, then expanded on the latter of the two through the next seven sentences and followed by an evaluation of the experience from the 8th through 53rd sentences. Interpreting this discrepancy between the seven participants in the extent to which blindness played a part in their responses, it appears as though for blind adults who have positive experiences with online learning, blindness plays an incidental role mixed in with the other factors such as content and course delivery. On the other hand, at least for these two individuals, a negative experience with online learning supersedes issues of blindness. Blindness was not the barrier. It therefore was entered late into the conversation of the informants. It did not matter that the participants were blind. It is reasonable to assume that the sighted learner would have had just as unfortunate an experience if enrolled in a noninteractive course or in attempting to enroll in an online course without computer proficiency and without technological guidance or supports.

Unlike blindness as a key referent within the phenomenological question, online learning with respect to technology or course delivery did not emerge as a salient category early within the responses. None of the respondents opened by commenting on course delivery and only one commented on delivery second. Three addressed delivery following two other topics.

The majority of respondents appeared to interpret the question—what is it like to be a blind online learner?—as evaluative, responding with an overall judgment of their experience. Five of the interviewees opened their first response in this way. Madeline, for example, said, "there were aspects of it I really liked and aspects of it I didn't like." Three of the respondents opened by naming or describing the content of their studies. The addition of opening the response with evaluation and with description derives the number of eight, rather than seven (the number of participants), because Bernice's initial response encompassed both evaluation and content. She said, "my experience with online learning probably is, it's a very positive experience because I did the online course with Norman Coombs and Dick Banks and it was how to—Barrier-free online learning for students with disabilities."

The course and/or program content [what the course was about e.g., cooking, adult learning] was analyzed according to how soon it was introduced as a topic by the participants. Content is of particular interest for two reasons. First, the study of content as a present or absent theme in phenomenological accounts of learners is important pedagogically. Ferrell, Persichitte, Lowell, and Roberts (2001) insist, "content determines methodology" (p. 603). Jardine, Clifford, and Friesen (2003) wrote about fostering content as the third leg of the stool. The other two legs are teachers and learners. Each member of the triad should support and inform the practice of the others. Yet the educational stool is often hobbled or even toppled by a weak content leg. The content is seldom permitted to inform how the learners should be taught.

The second reason why content is of particular interest in the phenomenological accounts of the learners is because Robinson (2000) wrote that the respondents in her research failed to introduce the course content as a topic of discussion. Coming full circle to the first section of this chapter that focussed on the relationship between the researcher and the participants, it must be noted that Robinson was a colleague of her research participants. She graduated from the same course of studies. Part of the reason that the informants did not introduce content as a topic of inquiry might have been that their interlocuter (Robinson) had a pre-established and assumed to be a shared understanding of the content. The topic might thereby have been considered to be a moot point. That being said, it is understandable that they did not introduce content as a discrete and substantial topic of conversation, but it is perhaps more revealing that Robinson's analysis also does not present them as incorporating content into the conversation about the way in which the course was delivered, nor their evaluation of the experience.

In the current research, three of the respondents addressed content in the first sentence. One respondent spoke of content in the 8th sentence, another in the 14th, and one in the 21st. The outlying response came at 54 sentences, still within the first two pages of transcripts.

Three plausible theories might explain the salience of content within the dialogue with blind online learners versus the absence of content as an emerging theme within Robinson's (2000) research with mainstream online learners. First, the notability or deviance might be in the absence of content within Robinson's research rather than with the references to content within the current research. This absence is in part explained above. In addition, the nature of Robinson's questions may not have elicited content themes amongst her respondents. There might have been attributes of her participants, characteristics of the program of study, or features of the delivery that muted mention of content. Robinson does not speculate on these conditions and wrote that she was surprised by the absence of content as topic implying that nonsalience of content within the accounts of graduates is common to online learning.

The other two theories therefore address the early and unmistakable emergence of content in the accounts of blind online learners as a unique occurrence within student accounts of online learning. One theory is that online learning, with its presentation of auditory and multiple simultaneous visual stimuli is overwhelming resulting in sensory and attentional overload. Mayer (2001) discussed the potential for overstimulation of receptive channels through poor practices in the design of multimedia. The theory, then, is that the sighted learners are overwhelmed by the multimedia nature of the online delivery such that they cannot concentrate on the content. Content for the blind learners, on the other hand, remains salient, because not receiving the visual stimuli means that they are not overstimulated in online learning.

This theory is countered on two accounts. First, none of the phenomenological accounts of what it is like to be a sighted online learner that were reviewed in this research including those of Dickie (1999), Hara and Kling (1999, 2000), and Robinson (2000) presented the experience of sensory overload in the accounts of their respondents. Second, the emergence of sensory overload theory derives from Mayer (2001) and several methodological flaws and questions emerge within his text. While Mayer reported empirically testing and supporting his propositions, he included minimal detail regarding these "experiments" neglecting to even state the sample size.

If accepted, Mayer's (2001) propositions imply bleak outcomes regarding the education of the blind. First, Mayer proposed that humans have two distinct yet complimentary learning channels, one of which receives and processes words and the other pictures. He wrote that the promise of multimedia learning comes in the interaction of the two channels. He continued that learning is deleteriously impacted by the common practice of text-only lessons. The blind, by virtue of not being able to see the pictures are excluded from one of the two channels of learning. Empirically, then, it should follow that blind learners perform significantly below their sighted peers in lessons that incorporate words and pictures. The high grades achieved by the participants in this research demonstrate that this is simply not the case.

Further, Mayer (2001) defined spatial ability as "the ability to generate, maintain, and manipulate mental visual images" (p. 172). People who are blind from birth or near-birth can be expected to have more difficulty generating mental visual images. Mayer implied that this further deleteriously impacts their learning potential. This is once again not evidenced in the learning outcomes of the current research respondents.

Mayer's (2001) propositions also fly in the face of the principles of universal design. Mayer's redundancy principle posits that only one visual and one auditory media be presented at one time. Specifically, his modality principle urges presentation of words in a multimedia message as spoken text rather than written text. In other words, an uncaptioned diagram would be synchronously accompanied by an auditory description. This is ineffective for deaf learners who would thereby not have access to an interpretation of the diagram. Universal design encourages planned redundancy of communication modes such that all learners have access to information.

Three pedagogical examples are used throughout Mayer's (2001) volume: (a) the formation of lightning storms, (b) the functioning of brakes, and (c) the functioning of pumps. Each one was taught as a concrete, sequential instructional module. Each has explicit binary conditions such as open and closed. Mayer used the three examples to illustrate the distinction between two theories of learning—information acquisition and knowledge construction. He propounded the latter. However, the three examples resonate with the former. The formation of lightning storms falls into the cognitive domain of learning. Operating brakes and pumps fall into the cognitive and psychomotor domains. None of the three examples draw upon the affective domain. It is in the affective domain of learning that emotional investment, and personal and shared meaning impact the construction of knowledge (Brooks & Brooks, 1999; Gardner, 1991; Goleman, 1994).

The third theory posed to explain why content was salient in the responses of the blind online learners in this research, whereas it was not in the responses of the sighted online learners in Robinson's (2000) research was corroborated by several of the respondents in the current research. Blind online learners usually have had multiple experiences of inaccessible education. Matthew's story in chapter 5 provided an extended example of a course in which he could not participate in the surveying assignments and thus received a failing grade. Teachers refer to blackboard illustrations or text that the blind student cannot see. Teachers direct students to spontaneously turn to pages in textbooks and read passages. The blind student usually receives a Braille equivalent weeks after the class has started, and the page numbers do not match in any case. Some blind learners cannot read the text at all, due largely to lack of teachers of Braille (Ferguson, 2001). Yet, the blind student learns the material. He has a lifetime of getting to the content beyond, or in spite of inaccessible educational technologies.

For the sighted learner, however, online learning is likely a first experience of inaccessible educational technologies. The inaccessible delivery is so forefront in the experience and recollection of online learning that content does not emerge as salient in phenomenological accounts. In regard to navigating educational technologies, blind learners might be positioned as what O'Connor (2000) calls "leading edge" and "early adopters" providing an example for the sighted. Ferrell, Persichitte, Lowell, and Roberts (2001) described an intriguing observation of their students—teachers of the visually impaired—

> the students reported that the distance learning experience brought them a new understanding of how children with visual impairments learn—and how much they relied on visual input when teaching—because now they, too, were not able to see the instructor or each other. (p. 603)

Conclusion of Chapter 8

The fourth stage of analysis of the transcripts of conversations with seven blind online learners focuses on discourse. How did the informants story their experiences as blind adults and as online learners? How did the relationship with the researcher impact those stories? Informed by practices of ethnographic research, a relationship of trust was nurtured between the interviewer and the research participants. The researcher's distance from the experience of being a blind online learner necessitated full accounts on the part of the informants.

The discursive constructions of responses to two open-ended questions posed to each of the seven participants informs the phenomenon of blind online learning. When asked to share whatever they chose of their life stories, the four Canadians opened with a description of their eye condition, whereas the three Americans did not. The posed hypothesis is that the American culture of blindness is such that a strong message of normality has been constructed by and about blind people. Blindness is just one characteristic of the person and a relatively unimportant characteristic at that. The Canadians, in absence of a strong voice of the organized blind, have not internalized the same message.

There were two main findings in analysis of the response to the question—what is it like to be a blind online learner. The first result is that five of the seven informants referred to the referent *blindness* early in their replies. The two exceptions were the respondents who had negative experiences of online learning. Their negative experiences were not a result of their blindness. Accordingly, blindness did not emerge as a factor in their responses to the questioning of their experiences.

The second result in analysis of the responses to the question—what is it like to be a blind online learner is that the informants took up the topic of the course content early and often within their responses. This emphasis differed from the findings of Robinson (2000) in her inquiry into what it is like to be a (sighted) online learner. Three theories were posed to explain this result, and two refuted. The first refuted theory is that the exceptional condition of interest was that the respondents in Robinson's study did not mention content, and not that the respondents in the current study did. The second refuted theory is that the sighted students experienced sensory and cognitive overload from the multimedia design of the online courses and thereby could not get to the content beyond the technology. By virtue of not being able to see, the blind students did not experience the overload. The third and supported theory is that blind students are used to inaccessible educational technologies and have experience in getting to the content not through, but in spite of the medium, whereas the sighted students are thwarted by this first experience of inaccessibility presented by the frustrating technologies of online learning. In this regard, the blind move to a position of "leading edge" for the sighted.

CHAPTER 9

CONCLUSIONS AND QUESTIONS FOR FURTHER INQUIRY

In order to inquire into the experience of online learning, five interactive interviews were conducted with adults who are totally blind and two interviews were conducted with adults who have low vision. The interview transcripts were analyzed using a quadri-reflexive framework (Alvesson & Sköldberg, 2000). In stage one of the analysis, each of the informants' biographical information and depiction of the experience of online learning were written up one-by-one and validated by the respective participant.

In stage two of the analysis, the seven depicted experiences were interpreted with respect to the three guiding research questions: (a) what is it like to be a blind online learner, (b) what are the best design characteristics of online learning, and (c) what is the impact of blind adults studying online. The interviews with the seven informants created a depiction of factors in the experience of online learning for blind students in answer to the first question. Probing what worked and did not work in the design of the courses and programs experienced by the informants contributed to design recommendations and supported the tips as presented by Coombs and Banks in answer to the second question. Themes emerged both from the literature and unprompted within the interviews concern-

Seeing Beyond Blindness, 175–187

ing the impact of online learning on the blind learners, on their student colleagues, on course design and instruction, and on public attitudes in answer to the third question.

Stage three of the analysis required revisiting the stories of the participants and their interpretations from a critical theoretical perspective. This analysis queried who were included as informants and who were excluded from the research. The social construction of attitudes about blindness was applied to determine what impact unconscious attitudes had on the depictions of blind online learners and on the research interpretations. Postman's (2003) questions regarding the sociological desirability of online learning were considered to query whether blind adults might benefit or suffer from engagement with this educational technology.

Stage four applied discourse analysis to the dramaturgical event of the interview (Berg, 1995) and to the interview transcripts. The analysis queried the effect that the actors in each interview (the informant and the researcher) and the relationship between them had on the research narratives. The responses to two open-ended questions were analyzed to interpret thematic salience and order. The two open-ended questions queried: (a) autobiographical information, and (b) what it is like to be a blind online learner.

Four main research interpretations emerged from the quadri-reflexive analysis. First, the depicted experiences of the seven informants indicated that online learning is possible, convenient, and prodigious for blind adults. Second, for the participants, online learning was experienced to its best advantage when it was simple, interactive, and accessible. Third, conditions that facilitated the informants' participation in online learning were access to and working knowledge of adaptive technologies as well as either a high level of technological proficiency or regular access to human supports. Fourth, course characteristics that were designed to benefit the blind learners in this research reportedly improved online learning for their sighted student colleagues.

Research Result One

Online Learning is Possible, Convenient and Prodigious for Blind Online Learners

At the basest level, this research asks whether it is even possible for blind adults to participate in online learning. At first glance, the participation of blind adults in online learning is counterintuitive. The almost exclusively visual design of computer interfaces is not amenable to blind users (National Research and Training Institute for the Blind, 2000).

However, neither is the face-to-face classroom designed for the blind. Bernice, one of the research informants, described the challenges posed by the reliance on blackboard illustrations and on-the-spot requests to turn to a certain page in a printed text. Marks (1999) explained that environments and practices were built for the sighted. In the case of online learning, the communication tools and content modules are primarily digital. In the case of face-to-face learning, a great deal of the communication is auditory, but the texts, assignments, and in-class illustrations are analogue. Negroponte (1995) explained that atoms are fixed in a single format whereas bits are easily manipulated and usable in multiple formats. In other words, the participation of blind adults in online learning may be more intuitive than participation in face-to-face classrooms provided that the blind users may manipulate the bits so that they are rendered in an accessible format.

All seven of the research informants experienced online learning as possible, and six of the seven carried through with the experience. One participant graduated from a postsecondary program in which the majority of the courses were online. Two participants were dedicated to postsecondary programs and had completed a number of online courses. Another participant was in the process of taking her third online course as a preprogram student. Her intention is to apply the courses toward a post-secondary program that is offered entirely online. Two participants had each completed one course online and were open to enrolling in future online courses. One participant successfully enrolled in an online course and then withdrew prior to participating. She expressed openness to enrolling in online courses in the future.

In reporting that online learning is possible, it was possible for each of the seven participants using adaptive technologies. JAWS screen reading software was used as the primary tool to facilitate accessibility by the five totally blind learners and by one of the learners with low vision. A synthesized voice read the words out loud to the users. The users had no need for a monitor unless they were sharing the computer with a sighted user. The seventh research participant, who has low vision, primarily used ZoomText screen enlarging software. The text and/or images are enlarged. The user must continually scan as only a portion of the screen fits into the view.

The advantage of online learning cited with the most frequency and emphasis by each of the seven research informants was its convenience. Convenience as operationally defined through conversations with the seven informants meant that the learners could study at a time, in a place, and at a pace that fit their busy lives. Four of the research participants are married and six have grown children and two have grandchildren. Five of the participants have full-time jobs that they maintained while studying.

These conditions might have been included in the profile of any group of online learners, and notably, Thompson (1998) found that this profile is common to online learners. When discussing the convenience factor, the informants in this research were speaking as online learners and not as blind adults. In other words, the convenience factor was only minimally associated with blindness. The participants' characteristic of blindness was only significant when blindness heightened other factors such as the length of time it took to travel to a postsecondary campus. Within the conversation, the factor of convenience superseded issues of blindness. The result of discussions regarding whether online learning would become a new type of segregated education for blind learners and whether students participating in online classrooms were forsaking an ambassadorial role for the blind was to conclude that the convenience of online learning is so advantageous that these other issues take a backseat.

Not only was online learning possible and convenient, for the research participants it was also prodigious. Madeline completed a master's degree that she would not have enrolled in if it had been only offered face-to-face. At the time of interview, Madeline's degree had already opened-up consulting opportunities. Currently, Madeline is beginning her second year as a certified teacher, and an interview with her employer indicates that she is a vital resource to their school board. Matthew and Sarah were in the process of completing master's degrees that they would not have considered if not for the online courses. Matthew spoke of personal growth through his program and career enhancement. Sarah formed international alliances that expanded her possibilities beyond her small community. Bernice and Sarah both perceived their career work enhanced through the content of their online courses.

Research Result Two

Three Essential Online Learning Characteristics—Simplicity, Interactivity, Accessibility

Coombs and Banks (2000) offered 16 tips for online learning. Fifteen of the 16 tips resonated with the content of the interview transcripts. The only tip that did not emerge within the research conversations recommended the instructor's setting of boundaries. The interviews were conducted with students and not instructors. Because boundaries did not emerge as a salient issue for the students, perhaps it can be postulated that the instructors handled the boundaries effectively.

The remaining 15 tips cluster into three overlapping categories. The categories are themselves included as tips. The three overarching tips are:

(a) keep it simple, (b) be interactive, and (c) be accessible. The other dozen tips are elaborations of these three central points.

Simplicity

With regard to simplicity, Coombs and Banks (2000) advise course designers to: (a) remember e-mail, (b) beware of techies, and (c) modularize. All six of the research participants who completed at least one online course experienced e-mail as effective, efficient, and uncomplicated. Each of the other communication tools were experienced by one or more of the participants as frustrating, and nonfunctional. These communication tools included: (a) bulletin boards, (b) voice-based chat, (c) text-based chat, and (d) simultaneous slide-show presentation with voice-based discussion. Coombs and Banks cautioned not to let those who are enamored with technology include tools that are complicated and unnecessary. Keeping it simple applies to the communication tools and the organization of the content. The research participants commended the course design when each of the learning units was clearly and explicitly available to the students. They did not have to search through layers of links in order to locate the next module.

Shannon did not experience the course enrollment interface as simple. She attempted clarification by cradling the telephone under her shoulder to talk to the course administrators while using her fingers to sign-in. She experienced multiple layers of links. She experienced the initial interface as so frustrating that she decided to suspend her experience at that point.

Interactivity

Coombs and Banks (2000) provided additional tips in elaboration of the higher-level tip to be interactive. They reminded readers that online learning is about people and not technology. The majority of the learners commented that they felt connected and part of a community of learners. Madeline expressed that the only time she felt isolated as a participant in online learning was when she was floundering in trying to use a bulletin board communication tool. As soon as the instructor reverted back to e-mail, Madeline felt that the course and her own contribution were back on course. Madeline and Matthew enthusiastically advocated for the blended model whereby students had concentrated-time study institutes between semesters of online learning. However, two of the other participants—Martin and Sarah—were not in blended model programs and yet perceived the courses as positively interactive. Martin is taking courses through a university that offers some of the courses face-to-face and others online. However, his experience differs from that of Madeline and Matthew in that Martin does not remain with the same cohort of learners in the same courses throughout his program. Through the use of communication tools, he experienced his online courses as interactive. Of her three online courses to date, Sarah most enjoyed the one that most facilitated interaction. She formed a strong alliance with a student colleague in another province and another living in Italy. They collaborated on assignments and on extracurricular learning.

Deborah was the only participant who completed an online course who did not experience it as interactive. While the course design met the first conditions of simplicity, it did not engage the learners. There was no communication between the learners, and very little between the learners and the instructors. Not coincidentally, Deborah was one of the two research participants who evaluated the experience negatively.

Coombs and Banks (2000) wrote that online learning is at its best advantage when it does not attempt to replicate the classroom. Deborah's course provided long lectures. The only distinction between this online design and the dispensary model of face-to-face teaching is that the online lectures were text-based. Deborah listened to them through the synthesized voice of her JAWS screen-reading software. In other words, she did not even have the aesthetic advantage of the human voice. One of the features most celebrated by the other research participants was the time-delayed interaction. Madeline, Matthew, Martin, Sarah, and Bernice each commented about the extensive online postings of the engaged students and their tendency to mull over the dialogue prior to contributing. The discussions were most engaging when the instructors were consistent with another of Coombs and Banks' tips—be a virtual host. Sarah experienced one instructor who was perhaps too reticent in contributing, to the extent that the postings took the dialogue in technologically excessive directions.

Accessibility

Moulton, Huyler, Hertz, and Levenson (2002) married the concepts of accessibility and usability. Online learning can be experienced as inaccessible if learners with sensory impairments such as blindness are unable to obtain the course content and unable to communicate with the instructor and student colleagues, including if the courseware is incompatible with the learners' adaptive technologies. Online learning can also be experienced as inaccessible if the learner cannot receive the course on his computer because of ineffective Internet connections, or if he cannot navigate the interface to get to the content modules or use the communication tools. O'Connor (2000) wrote that people with disabilities are taking the leading edge in online learning. Blind learners have experienced a lifetime of inaccessibility. They have been unable to read what the teacher is writing on the blackboard, and usually have to wait well into the course prior to receiving a Braille version of the text. For most sighted learners, online learning may pose a first experience of inaccessibility. In the analysis of this research, it is theorized that the course content was salient for the blind learners in their description of what it is like to be a blind online learner whereas it was not for the learners in Robinson's (2000) research with (sighted) online learners, because blind learners are used to getting to the content in spite of the educational technologies whereas sighted learners are not. In other words, sighted online learners can learn from the experience of blind online learners. The phenomenologically blind can lead the virtually blind.

Coombs and Banks (2000) provided six tips to enhance accessibility. First, make the course design a team project. While none of the learners in this research were asked what would enhance accessibility during the design phase of the course, several of the instructors asked the learners' advice during the course, and several participants volunteered advice for the design of their next courses. Second, it is recommended that online courses be designed for universal access. All students should be able to access the information and participate in the communication. One means of facilitating universal access is recommended in the third tip—provide redundant communication modes. None of the research participants experienced equivalent content provided in alternate modes such as audio and text. Each of them would welcome that option if available.

Coombs and Banks' (2000) fourth accessibility tip is to understand the problems of students with disabilities. Each of the learners in this research was enrolled in a mainstream program. To their knowledge, it was the first time that the instructors had taught blind students. The instructors were unaware of the need to distribute text-based materials well in advance of the course start-date so that the blind student could have the text translated into Braille. As a result of engaging with the blind students, the instructors were in compliance with Coombs and Banks' fifth accessibility tip that is to have a system to deal with special problems. The administrators at Sarah's institution put a red star beside her name as a reminder to send the materials out in advance.

The sixth and final tip to facilitate accessibility is to understand adaptive technologies. Deborah is sceptical about the complete universal design of online courses. She said that even if the lectures were provided as an audio link to a human voice she would still require her screen reading software to identify and locate the link. In addition, if the universal design feature were a built-in screen reader with a synthesized voice, then she would rather use her own screen reading software with which she is already familiar. If adaptive technologies are not going to become obsolete, then it is important that course designers are aware of compatibility issues. For example, JAWS screen reading software cannot voice describe images or icons unless the designer has inserted an alt-tag or long-description attribute, or in other words, a text-based version of the image.

Research Result Three

Adaptive Technologies, and Technological Proficiency or Human Supports

As described above, online learning was experienced as possible by all of the informants in this research. However, online learning would not have been possible without the use of adaptive technologies. Each of the participants would have experienced the courses as inaccessible without the technology. The participants used a variety of adaptive technologies, the most common of which was JAWS screen-reading software. This condition excludes numerous prospective students from the experience of online learning. Prospective students who cannot afford the adaptive technologies cannot participate in online learning. Madeline shared that her office contained approximately $25,000 of computer equipment. Admittedly, Madeline had more adaptive technologies than are absolutely necessary, but the JAWS software package alone costs approximately $1,100. Having JAWS alone without other adaptive technologies does not allow for Braille embossing, or portability of information. The research participants also shared that there are limited opportunities for advanced training in the use of computer and adaptive technologies. Specialized training is expensive, and generic training is often uninformative.

In other words, for the participants in this research, access to and knowledge of adaptive technologies was necessary but not sufficient. Martin, Bernice, and Deborah are technologically proficient. They provide computer training as part of their career work. Madeline and Sarah both have technologically proficient husbands who assist them with online learning and the use of their adaptive technologies. Matthew has regular access to a past colleague who works in information technologies (IT) and works out of a neighboring building. The only participant who was neither technologically proficient nor had regular access to human computer supports was Shannon. She withdrew from the course following the frustrating enrolment phase.

Research Result Four

Course Characteristics Designed to Benefit Blind Learners Improve Online Learning for All Students

Coombs and Banks (2000) described electronic curb-cuts. Curb-cuts are the portion of the sidewalk that rests flush with the road. They were designed for people in wheelchairs. However, curb-cuts are more commonly used by mothers with strollers, cyclists, and inline skaters. Likewise, computer applications have been designed for people with disabilities. Coombs and Banks (personal communication, March 19, 2003) used the example of the scanner. The scanner was very expensive when used strictly by people with disabilities who needed materials in a digital format. When scanners came into popular use by Web designers and then the general public who wanted to post digital photographs, the price dropped dramatically.

Several of the participants in this research experienced electronic curb-cuts. Madeline could not use the bulletin board. She thought that her blindness was the interfering factor. As one member in a class of eight, Madeline was a significant member of the class. The instructor stopped using the bulletin board and reverted back to e-mail. Madeline reported that the entire class celebrated. The others were not able to use the bulletin board either.

Matthew has low vision. He asked that the instructor and students use a san-serif font such as Arial, as the little lines decorating the characters in fonts such as Times New Roman interfered with clarity. He also asked that they used a larger size font and be wary of colors that are difficult to distinguish. Some of Matthew's colleagues, many of whom are mature students and have multiple commitments such as family and work that leave them tired at the end of the day when they read their e-mail also commented that they benefited from Matthew's requests.

Sarah had a frustrating experience in one of her classes in which a few members of the class were enthusiastic computer users. They began to take the bulletin board in technologically excessive directions, requesting that the students use links, graphic design, and other such features. Sarah was already experiencing the bulletin board as inaccessible and was reliant upon her husband to read the postings out to her. Sarah made the decision to disclose that she has low vision and express her frustration. The students returned to appropriate use of the bulletin board. Several of the students who were not technologically proficient were also experiencing panic at the new technological demands and celebrated the return to appropriate use of the bulletin board. Sarah formed two strong alliances with student colleagues as a result.

Questions for Further Inquiry

Impact

While most of the informants shared that they benefited through online learning, this research still leaves the third guiding question regarding impact largely unanswered. Kim-Rupnow, Dowrick, and Burke (2001) posed the question—"Do the increase in distance education programs and use of advanced technology indicate better access and better outcomes in higher education for persons with disabilities" (p. 25). The participants in this research expressed that the digital content modules were more accessible than the paper texts of face-to-face classrooms. Five of the six also indicated that they would not have been able to participate in the courses and/or programs of study unless offered partly or entirely online. The outcomes for the participants at the time of interview were also positive overall. Madeline graduated with a master's degree. She is now a certified teacher. Matthew and Sarah will graduate with a master's degree in the foreseeable future. Martin will graduate with a bachelor's degree. These are four degrees that the informants claim would not have been earned if the respective programs of study did not have online courses. Bernice and Deborah learned information and made career applications that they would not have had access to through face-to-face delivery.

While these achievements predict positive impact for blind learners overall, the question of educational outcomes might best be answered through alternate research methods. As summarized by Huebner and Wiener (2001), it is not known, however, how effective the application of [online] learning is to the education and rehabilitation of individuals who are visually impaired" (p. 520). Analysis of statistics of post-secondary student enrolment and graduation would address questions such as: (a) are enrolment, course completion and program graduation rates of blind adults increasing over time; (b) what percentage of blind postsecondary students are enrolling in online courses and/or programs; and (c) is there a statistical difference between face-to-face and online course completion and program graduation rates of blind adults. Transition to employment and career enhancement might also be analyzed using a large sample.

Postsecondary Students with Disabilities

In order to qualify for participation in this research, informants were to be legally blind. Blindness was an intuitive research starting point in inquiring into the online experiences of students with disabilities because the computer interface is primarily visual. It would now be informative for prospective students, course instructors and designers, and post-secondary administrators to access research on what it is like to be an online learner with other types of disabling conditions. Do deaf students experience inaccessibility of online content modules and/or communication tools? What design characteristics best meet the needs of students with learning disabilities? Can plain language interpretation be designed into online courses for students with cognitive impairments? What adaptive technologies are required by learners with physical disabilities? Most important, how can the principles of universal design be applied to online learning so that each course and program meets the needs of all students without the need for retrofitting or accommodation?

Multidimensional Learning

Mayer's (2001) theory of multimedia learning was critiqued in chapter 8 largely due to: (a) the design of the empirical research presented in support of the theory; and (b) propositions that do not hold when applied to blind learners, such as the statement that learners who do not have access to both textual and pictorial content achieve poorer learning outcomes. However, Mayer's research made multimedia course design salient. His theory raises issues warranting further inquiry at the intersection of blindness and learning, and particularly online learning with its capacity for text, sound, narration and animation. Some of these questions warranting further inquiry are:

- Are mental pictures equivalent to visual pictures and if so, is the use of metaphor effective in educational contexts? Are metaphors predominantly visual or can they be equivalently interpreted through other senses?;
- How paramount is experience to reception of visual images? If images are often and fully described to a blind child, are his experiences of educational images different than for someone who did not receive this description? If so, in what way?;
- It has been suggested that blind people may better attain and retain focus, because with the absence of visual stimuli, they are less prone to what Mayer presented as the capacity-limitation hypothesis (p. 152), or in other words, sensory and even cognitive overload. Can this be empirically substantiated?;
- Where do images described in words "fit" in terms of multimedia cognitive theory? Are they words or are they pictures? Are binary communication channels an accurate depiction?;

- Because we mediate the world through words (Magee & Milligan, 1995), or in other words, language is propositional, are the experiences of blind people essentially the same as the sighted?
- Is there a difference in terms of cognitive processing between reading text on the computer monitor and hearing it through screen reading software?

Personal Closing Note From the Researcher

I would like to close this depiction of the research by sharing the highlights of what I learned and where I will take the research from here. This is a vital and imperative component of research that is often forgotten. Throughout the research—in choosing a topic and then framing questions; while collecting data such as through interviewing; underlying interpretation, and; in writing and verbally presenting, discussing, and defending the research—it is vital to ask the same question in two different ways. First, what matters about this research? Second, so what? If we cannot answer these two questions, at least for ourselves as we go about the course of our lives, then we must take another look at our research and re-examine whether it is worth doing and why.

A humorous fictional account of masturbatory academia is presented by Alexander McCall Smith (2004b) in *Portuguese Irregular Verbs*, *The Finer Points of Sausage Dogs* (2004c), and *At the Villa of Reduced Circumstances* (2004a). The novels present the misadventures and foibles of the pompous Dr. von Igelfeld, a professor of romance philology. His posturing and disdain for others leads him unawares into comedic encounters, such as when he was mistaken for a respected leading professor of veterinary medicine—Igelfold—and sent from his German homeland to Arkansas where he delivered an address on sausage dogs and then was trapped into conducting veterinary surgery, whereupon he caused the amputation of three of a sausage dog's legs (two of which were perfectly functional).

In pondering *so what* with regards to the research presented in this text, with respect to online learning, I have been de-dazzled by the intrigue of new educational technologies. I believe that the key principles of universal design of online learning are simplicity, interactivity, and accessibility. In short, this means: (a) dividing content into digestible learning modules, (b) mailing-out large data files in multimodal formats on CD-ROM, and (c) promoting critical inquiry by following up each learning module with moderated interaction through grouped e-mails. This is a shift in practice for me. Prior to this research I was a vocal advocate for learning moderation systems and particularly the bulletin board communication tool. Speaking from experience as I am currently teaching online (to sighted postsecondary students), working off of learning moderation systems puts the focus back on the course content and critical thinking, and as a result, the technology mostly disappears into the background. So now I hope to convince others to make the same change and help them to do so through dissemination of information. In terms of further research, I have been interviewing blind and sighted learners from Kindergarten through postsecondary to explore the design of technology-infused classrooms and lectures supplemented by Web sites and online communication tools. The main question driving this research is which designs are accessible and interactive. Consistent with the research depicted in this text, the answer rests primarily in simplicity.

In addition to applying my research to shifting practices in online learning, I have assimilated beliefs and attitudes about blindness to construct new personal meanings through spending time and having many conversations with blind adults. I now truly believe that while not being able to see is a nuisance, blindness should be perceived as a barrier to very little. Blind adults who have been supported to believe and trust in themselves and to learn Braille, orientation and mobility, and functional adult living skills such as cooking and home maintenance, through organizations such as the Louisiana Center for the Blind (LCB), are independent, self-empowered, confident citizens. I have had the pleasure of meeting many adults for whom this description can be applied. In terms of further research, I plan to further explore empowerment through education by conducting interpretive research with blind parents, blind postsecondary students and with blind school children. I hope to add to the emerging body of literature that is (as so concisely stated by LCB)—changing what it means to be blind.

CHAPTER 10

THE IMPORTANCE OF REFLEXIVITY IN BLINDNESS RESEARCH

This text sought to position blindness within the periodic cultural construct of Middle America. As such, the dominant role of visual aesthetics was explicated. While the period of *modernism*, with its respect and concordance with dominant authority and thus the imperative of fixed codes of practice, and then *postmodernism* as a sometimes resistant and sometimes reactionary approach to this authority and monoliths, were initially acted out by the subversive minority, this is no longer the case. While the words "modernism" and "post-modernism" may not be in the public vernacular, the practiced fall-out from cultural consciousness are pervasive. In his chapter, "Postmodernism and Consumer Society," Jameson (1998) wrote that the most telling evidence of a widespread periodic shift is when the principles are applied and taught within the social mold of the school and post-secondary institution. The status quo is no longer critiqued and subverted by a group of rabble-rousers. It is adopted and established in the mainstream academy. "For another, the classics of high modernism are now part of the so-called canon and are taught in schools and universities—-which at once empties them of any of their older subversive power" (p. 143). I argue that in the 8 years since publication of the text in which Jameson's chapter appeared—*The Anti-Aesthetic: Essays on Postmodern Cul-*

Seeing Beyond Blindness, 189–193

ture, postmodernism has also become established public discourse. Postmodernist titles are now assigned textbooks and the tenets debated within seminars.

With respect to capitalism, consumerism, and the objectification of the body, the public at one and the same time practices its corollaries and is aware of and even voices the objections, that is, tsk-tsking the televised beauty pageant watched on the huge flat-screen television from the comfort of a leather couch. Jameson enumerated the signposts of modernism.

> New types of consumption; planned obsolescence; an ever more rapid rhythm of fashion and styling changes; the penetration of advertising, television and the media generally to a hitherto unparalleled degree throughout society; the replacement of the old tension between city and country, center and province, by the suburb and by universal standardization; the growth of the great networks of superhighways and the arrival of automobile culture--these are some of the features which would seem to mark a radical break with that older prewar society in which high modernism was still an underground force. (p. 143)

None of these features have become obselete. Families have more expendable income than ever before. Wardrobes have modified and mushroomed well beyond the limits of utility. Fashion means excess and *nonsense*. Winter weather is greeted by bare midriffs and high heels. Middle America's favorite passtime is shopping, evidenced by the inability to find parking in the mall lot on any given Saturday. Christmas advertising begins in September or earlier, flanked by the imperative for back-to-school costumes and accessories signifying "attitude."

Parents are hard-pressed to find any Christmas toy that their child does not already have. Smart marketers plan an annual collection to ensure brand loyalty. Barbie and her entourage were heavily marketed as "she" starred in recreations of *The Nutcracker Suite*, *Rapunzel*, and *Swan Lake*, followed up by more glitter and girl-appeal with their own creations of *Fairytopia* and *The Magic of Pegasus*. As well as the movie on DVD and video platforms, each set (items sold separately) comes with three to six different Barbie figurines, a pair of horses with a carriage, a castle and other accessories, as well as life-size costumes, crowns, wings, and wands. In 2005, *The Magic of Pegasus* movie was released in the summer rather than waiting until closer to Christmas, so that the children with contemporary absence of delayed gratification would already own the movie and several of the trappings and the parents would be freed to purchase the remaining for Christmas.

While parents are purchasing such toys to excess, it is not without guilt. We are aware of consumerism and its fallout. We fret about spoiled children and overflowing garbage dumps. We absolve our guilt by sponsoring children in third-world countries and increasing other charitable donations. Yet, we do not stop buying. Advertising trailers on *The Magic of Pegasus* have already prepared the girls for the upcoming *Barbie Diaries* and *Mermaidia*. Christmas sales in 2006 and 2007 will soar as these items clear the toy store shelves in droves. While the surface meaning of consumerism is available to conscious awareness, the corollaries run deeper. The entangled web of postmodern crisis is largely unconscious and thus all the more powerful.

The meaning of consumerism has shifted. When the *Random House Dictionary* published its updated edition in 1980, "consumerism" was defined as "a movement for the protection of the consumer against inferior or dangerous products, misleading advertising, etc." This particular movement has been activated. The time dedicated to disclaimers and cautions on television advertisements for pharmaceuticals and diet products often matches or exceeds time for promotion. The new definition of consumerism is part of common vernacular, only this time it is not a movement. In 2005, Wikipedia, the online dictionary/encyclopedia defines "consumerism" as "a term used to describe the effects of equating personal happiness with purchasing material possessions and consumption." Except for a subversive minority, people do not particularly want to change the status quo of material goods, even while they are aware of its deleterious consequences.

While the general public and academics alike are generally versed in consumerism, the first chapter of this text presented the deficiencies in the knowledge base. What has been scantily inquired into, is the link between consumerism and vision. Consumerism rests on an appeal to the visual. Although critiqued, Maslow's (1943) hierarchy of needs is an explanatory model in this case. Twenty-first century Middle Americans have their basic needs for food, water, and shelter met. If someone does not have relationships to satisfy their social needs, he can purchase the company of others or go online for virtual friendships. So instead of ascending to self-actualization, we, as a culture, have instead adopted the opposite. With our basic and even secondary needs met, we spend our money on visual titillation. We have become visio-centric.

The consequence for the blind is stigma. The sighted population cannot fathom being without the gateway to the vision-centered cultural arena. How could we exist without vision? To not see the expressions on our childrens' faces, to not see the colors of the sunset, to not participate in the home décor revolution is perceived as a tragedy. The consequence is that blind persons are pitied, feared, or awed. Whichever the reaction, the positioning of blind persons is that of "the other." Without belonging to the grand narrative club of vision, the blind are ostracized. They are not perceived as normal human beings.

Social science research cannot inquire into subjects of blindness, or for that matter engage blind subjects as research *participants*, without recognizing the visio-centric nature of twenty-first century Middle America. Postmodernity shatters the academic's belief in representation. In modern conceptions of research, the primary role of the researcher was to represent—to cast his gaze upon subjects and to paint a picture, create an image, of their experience. To represent, one must see and then create a reproduction of that sight for others. Seeing was privileged as the route to knowledge. Objectivity and replicability were practiced. Postmodernity de-throned the objective gaze and the de-sanctioned researchers from *representing*.

The most dire consequence of modern approaches to research was the misrepresentation and thus the silencing or muting of the subjects. For the purposes of intellectual intrigue, the research subjects are usually those outside the dominant norm. Those conducting the research were not particularly interested in representing the dominant—middle class, educated persons of European descent. The outcome holds no intrigue and besides, the sighted can see for themselves by peering out their own windows; there is no need for representation. So who were the research subjects? The others such as the blind. The blind, who could not *see* to *represent* in the manner of the sighted, and who made it into the academy in tiny numbers through the hegemony of the sighted educational constructions, do not have the mechanism to speak for themselves. And what of those who were speaking for the blind? Owens (1998) wrote that the representative voice served to repress.

> Despite his or her benevolence in representing those who have been denied access to the means of representation, the [researcher] inevitably functions as an agent of the system of power that silenced these people in the first place. Thus, they are twice victimized: first by society, and then by the [researcher] who presumes the right to speak on their behalf. (p. 79)

All research is designed, developed, enacted, and *applied* based on interpretation. Those interpretations are constructed by the time and place culture of the researchers and of the research participants offering up the cultural collusions for researcher interpretation. It is imperative that we see blindness through the lens of visio-centrism. Unless we are aware that we are living in a culture of visual predilection, the way in which we frame our questions, the way in which we design our "experiments," and the way in which we engage participation and interpret the meaning of the interlocution will be highly biassed and/or meaningless. Blind people are the "other" in a material culture of sight. As a sighted majority we design situations that make sense to a person with vision. With our disbelief that people can happily exist without vision, our protesting ears cannot hear deeper conversation beyond. All of this needs to be taken into consideration when researching in the field of blindness.

Returning now to the question above—How could we exist without vision—the methodological response is to inquire into the experience and perception of those who do live without vision. Research into blindness gives us great insight into the experience of vision. As has been argued, understanding the role of vision in our contemporary consciousness and unconscious construction of our social world is paramount.

Interpretive research into blindness is imperative. Reflexive positioning catalyzes a social constructionist awareness and thus makes visual predilection and visio-centrism accountable in blindness research. Beyond visio-centrism, interpretive research is also critical of other cultural collusions. Reflexive awareness leaves no domain as sacred. It calls the discourse, power affiliations, and relationships into question. Interpretive researchers recognize that we have constructed the social world that we live in and that this social world is not fixed. The institutions we have erected and social practices we have reified can be changed. Research practices are no more sacred and sanctified than any other social constructions. The blind person's cultural positioning as the "other" means that they have largely been (mis)represented by those with sight. Further, blind personhood is often left out of the research entirely, with a dehumanizing focus on technology, biomechanics, and rehabilitation.

Interactive conversations highlight personal voice, and iterative interpretation in conjunction with blind persons themselves. Interpretive research topples the authority and privilege of single methods, meaning that postmodern pastiches of approaches can be designed in response to the particular research questions. Interpretive research into blindness facilitates a new perspective on vision and allows blind people to take up their own experience and assume their rightful place as informed knowers.

REFERENCES

Alvesson, M., & Sköldberg, K. (2000). *Reflexive methodology: New vistas for qualitative research.* Thousand Oaks, CA: Sage.

Asch, A. (1995, November). Visual impairment and blindness [Electronic version]. *The Braille Monitor,* 38-52.

Aspland, T. (1999). A research journey: Struggling with the evolution of a methodological pastiche. *Education Research and Perspectives, 26*(2), 105-126.

Barasch, M. (2001). *Blindness: The history of a mental image in western thought.* New York: Routledge.

Berg, B. L. (1995). *Qualitative research methods for the social sciences.* Toronto, Canada: Allyn & Bacon.

Blaser, A. (2001, September). Distance learning—boon or bane? *Ragged Edge Online.* Retrieved September 9, 2002, from http://www.raggededgemagazine.com

Boman, S. (2002). *Ex-sighted, a new vision.* Ponoka, Alberta, Canada: Skillion.

Boshier, R., & Mun Onn, C. (2000). Discursive constructions of Web learning and education. *Journal of Distance Education, 15*(2), 1-16.

Brambring, M., & Troster, H. (1994, Jan/Feb). The assessment of cognitive development in blind infants and preschoolers. *Journal of Visual Impairment and Blindness, 88*(1), 9-19.

Brooks, J., & Brooks, M. (1999). *In search for understanding: The case for constructivist classrooms.* Alexandria, VA: Association for Supervision and Curriculum Development.

Burgstahler, S. (2003, March). *Developing policy for making distance learning programs accessible to everyone.* Paper presented at the 2003 Technology and Persons with Disabilities Conference. Retrieved May 8, 2003, from http://www.csun.edu/cod/conf/2003/proceedings/137.htm

Burgstahler, S. (2002). *Real connections: Making distance learning accessible to everyone.* Unpublished manuscript, University of Washington, DO-IT.

Burgstahler, S. (2002). Universal design of distance learning. *Information Technology and Disabilities, 8*(1). Retrieved May 8, 2003, from http://www.rit.edu/~easi/ itd/itdv08n1/burgstahler.htm

Burgstahler, S. (2002). *Universal design of instruction.* Unpublished manuscript, University of Washington DO-IT.

Cappelli, G. (2003). E-learning in the postsecondary education market: A view from Wall Street. In M. S. Pittinsky (Ed.), *The wired tower: Perspectives on the impact of the Internet on higher education* (pp. 41-63). Upper Saddle River, NJ: Financial Times Prentice Hall.

Chandler, J., Hu, D., Arndt, K., White, J., & Smith, V. (2002, June). *The beyondcompliance coordinating committee: Reconceptualizing disability at Syracuse University.* Paper presented at the Second City Conference on Disability Studies and Education, Chicago.

Clark, R. E., & Estes, F. (1999, March-April). The development of authentic educational technologies. *Educational Technology,* 5-16.

Cook, R. A., & Gladhart, M. A. (2002). A survey of online instructional issues andstrategies for postsecondary students with learning disabilities. *Information Technology and Disabilities, 8*(1). Retrieved May 8, 2002, from http://www.rit.edu/~easi/itd/itdv08n1/cook_gladhart.htm

Coombs, N., & Banks, R. (2000, March). *Distance learning and students with disabilities: Easy tips for teachers.* Paper presented at the 2000 Technology and Persons with Disabilities Conference. Retrieved May 8, 2003, from http://www.csun.edu/cod/conf/2000/proceedings/0119Coombs.htm

Dickie, S. (1999). *The lived experience of being a distance learner.* Unpublished master's thesis, Athabasca University, Canada.

Dossa, P. (1990). Women and disability: The myth of the autonomous individual. *Journal of Practical Approaches to Developmental Handicap, 14*(2), 37-42.

Dreyfus, H. (2001). *On the Internet: Thinking in action.* New York: Routledge.

Ellis, C., Kiesinger, C., & Tillman-Healy, L. (1997). Interactive interviewing: Talking about emotional experience. In R. Hertz (Ed.), *Reflexivity and voice* (pp. 119-149). Thousand Oaks, CA: Sage.

Emerson, R. M., Fretz, R. I., & Shaw, L. L. (1995). *Writing ethnographic fieldnotes.* Chicago: University of Chicago Press.

Ferguson, R. J. (Ed.). (2001). *We know who we are: A history of the blind in challenging educational and socially constructed policies: A study in policy archeology.* San Francisco: Caddo Gap.

Ferrell, K. A. (1996). Your child's development. In M. C. Holbrook (Ed.), *Children with visual impairments: A parents' guide* (pp. 73-96). Bethesda, MD: Woodbine House.

Ferrell, K. A., Persichitte, K. A., & Lowell, N. L. (2000, March). *Distance learning technologies for blind and visually impaired students.* Paper presented at the 2000 Technology and Persons with Disabilities Conference. Retrieved May 8, 2003, from http://www.csun.edu/cod/conf2000/proceedings/gensess_proceedings. html

Ferrell, K. A., Persichitte, K. A., Lowell, N., & Roberts, S. (2001). The evolution of a distance delivery system that supports content, learners, and pedagogy. *Journal of Visual Impairment & Blindness, 95,* 597-608.

Fetterman, D. M. (1998). *Ethnography* (2nd ed.). Thousand Oaks, CA: Sage.

Foucault, M. (1972). *The archaeology of knowledge.* (Tavistock Publications, Ltd., Trans.). London: Routledge (Original work published 1969)

Foucault, M. (1972-1977). *Power/knowledge: Selected interviews and other writings.* (C. Gordon, Ed.). New York: Pantheon.

Franklin, U. M. (1999). *The real world of technology* (Rev. ed.). Toronto, Ontario, Canada: House of Anansi.

French, S., & Swain, J. (2001). The relationship between disabled people and health and welfare professionals. In G. L. Albrecht, K. D. Seelman, & M. Bury (Eds.), *Handbook of disability studies* (pp. 734-753). Thousand Oaks, CA: Sage.

Friesen, N. (2002). Is there a body in this class? In M. van Manen (Ed.), *Writing in the dark: Phenomenological studies in interpretive inquiry* (pp. 221-236). London, Ontario, Canada: Althouse.

Gadamer, H. G. (1999). *Truth and method.* (J. Weinsheimer & D. G. Marshall, Trans.) New York: Continuum. (Original work published 1960)

Gardner, H. (1991). *The unschooled mind: How children think & how schools should teach.* New York: Basic Books.

Garrison, D. R., & Anderson, T. (2003). *E-Learning in the 21st century: A framework for research and practice.* New York: RoutledgeFalmer.

Goffman, E. (1963). *Stigma: Notes on the management of spoiled identity.* Englewood Cliffs, NJ: Prentice Hall.

Goffman, E. (1959). *The presentation of self in everyday life.* Garden City, NY: Anchor Books.

Goleman, D. (1994). *Emotional intelligence*. Bantam, New York.

Habermas, J. (1972). *Knowledge and human interest.* London: Heinemann.

Hacking, I. (1999). *The social construction of what?* Cambridge, MA: Harvard University Press.

Hamilton, E. (1942). *Mythology: Timeless tales of gods and heroes*. New York: Warner.

Hara, N., & Kling, R. (2000). Students' distress with a Web-based distance education course: An ethnographic study of participants' experiences. *Indiana University, Centre for Social Infomatics.* Retrieved September 18, 2002, from http:// www. slis.indiana.edu/CSI/Wp/wp00-01B.html

Hara, N., & Kling, R. (1999). Students' frustrations with a web-based distance education course. *First Monday, 4*(12). Retrieved September 18, 2002, from http:// firstmonday.org/issues/issue4_12/hara/index.html

Haraway, D. (1998, Fall). Situated knowledges: The science question in feminism and the privilege of partial perspective. *Feminist Studies, 14*(3), 575-599.

Hartin, P. (2000, November). *Is it time to start thinking unitary: Consumers and service providers—a vital partnership.* Paper presented at the World Blind Union General Assembly, Melbourne, Australia.

Herrmann, D. (1998). *Helen Keller: A life.* New York: Alfred A. Knopf.

Heidegger, M. (1977). *Basic writings.* (D. Krell, Ed.). New York: Harper & Row.

Heshusius, L. (2003, June). *A life long struggle in special education with the other, theory,the self, other difficult things.* Paper presented at the Second City Conference on Disability Studies and Education, Chicago.

Huebner, K. M., & Wiener, W. R. (2001). Editorial. *Journal of Visual Impairment and Blindness, 95*(9), 515-517.

Jameson, F. (1998). Postmodernism and consumer society. In H. Foster (Ed.), *The anti-aesthetic: Essays on postmodern culture* (pp. 127-144). New York: New Press.

Jardine, D. W., Clifford, P., & Friesen, S. (2003). *Back to the basics of teaching and learning: Thinking the world together.* London: Erlbaum.

Jernigan, K. (1965). Blindness—concepts and misconceptions. *Braille Monitor,* 76-85.

Jernigan, K. (1990). Blindness—handicap or characteristic. In F. Matson (Ed.), *Walking alone and marching together: A history of the organized blind movement in the United States,* 1950-1990 (pp. 176-186). Baltimore: National Federation of the Blind. (Reprinted from unpublished manuscript, 1963)

Junefelt, K. (2004). Identity and development: Lessons learned from a blind child. *Top Language Disorders, 24*(3), 187-199.

Kim-Rupnow, W. S., Dowrick, P. W., & Burke, L. S. (2001). Implications for improving access and outcomes for individuals with disabilities in post-secondary distance education. *The American Journal of Distance Education, 15*(1), 25-40.

Kinash, S. (2003, March). *Questioning online learning for blind post-secondary students.* Paper presented at the 2003 Technology and Persons with Disabilities Conference. Retrieved May 8, 2003, from http://www.csun.edu/cod/conf/2003/proceedings/152.htm

Kinash, S. (2002, June). *Online education in disability studies, and interactive interviewing online as research methodology.* Paper presented at the Second City Conference on Disability Studies and Education, Chicago.

Kincheloe, J. L., & Berry, K. S. (2004). *Rigour and complexity in educational research: Conceptualizing the bricolage.* Berkshire, England: Open University Press.

Kvam, M. H. (2005). Experiences of childhood sexual abuse among visually impaired adults in Norway: Prevalence and characteristics. *Journal of Visual Impairment and Blindness, 99*(1), 5-14.

Levine, A. (2003). Higher education: A revolution externally, evolution internally. In M. S. Pittinsky (Ed.), *The wired tower: Perspectives on the impact of the Internet on higher education* (pp. 13-39). Upper Saddle River, NJ: Financial Times Prentice Hall.

Levtzion-Korach, O., Tennenbaum, A., Schnitzer, R., & Ornoy, A. (2000). Early motor development of blind children. *Journal of Paediatric Child Health 36,* 226-229.

Magee, B., & Milligan, M. (1995). *On blindness.* New York: Oxford.

Marks, D. (1999). *Disability: Controversial debates and psychosocial perspectives.* New York: Routledge.

Marshall, C., & Rossman, G. (1989). *Designing qualitative research.* Newbury Park, CA: Sage.

Maslow, A. (1943). A theory of human motivation. *Psychological Review, 50,* 370-396. Retrieved April 06, 2006, from http://psychclassics.yorku.ca/Maslow/motivation.htm.

Mayer, R. E. (2001). *Multi-media learning.* New York: Cambridge.

McCall Smith, A. (2004a). *At the villa of reduced circumstances.* Toronto, Canada: Vintage.

McCall Smith, A. (2004b). *Portuguese irregular verbs.* Toronto, Canada: Vintage.

McCall Smith, A. (2004c). *The finer points of sausage dogs.* Toronto, Canada: Vintage.

McGrane, S. (2000). *CNET Special reports: Is the Web truly accessible to the disabled?* Retrieved May 29, 2004, from http://www.cnet.com/specialreports/ 0-6014-7-1530073.html

McLuhan, M. (1964). *Understanding media: The extensions of man.* New York: McGraw-Hill.

McNamee, L., & Roberts, T. S. (2002, July). Online collaborative learning in a tertiary environment. In S. McNamara & E. Stacey (Eds.), *Untangling the Web: Establishing learning links.* Melbourn, Australia: ASET Conference Proceedings. Retrieved from http://www.aset.org.au/confs/2002/mcnamee.html

Merriam, S. B. (1998). *Qualitative research and case study applications in education.* San Francisco: Jossey-Bass.

Mills, S. (1997). *Discourse.* New York: Routledge.

Monbeck, M. E. (1973). *The meaning of blindness: Attitudes toward blindness and blind people.* Bloomington: Indiana University Press.

Montgomery-Whicher, R. (2002). Drawing to attention. In M. van Manen (Ed.), *Writing in the dark: Phenomenological studies in interpretive inquiry* (pp. 28-48). London, Ontario, Canada: Althouse.

Moulton, G., Huyler, L., Hertz, J., & Levenson, M. (2002). *Accessible technology in today's business: Case studies for success.* Redmond, WA: Microsoft.

Moustakas, C. (1994). *Phenomenological research methods.* Thousand Oaks, CA: Sage.

Murdoch, H. (1994, July/August). The development of infants who are deaf-blind: A case study. *Journal of Visual Impairment and Blindness, 88*(4), 357-368.

National Research and Training Institute for the Blind. (2000, February). Technology. *The Braille Monitor, 43*(2). Retrieved September 20, 2002, from http:// www.nfb.org/bm/ bm0002/brlm0002.htm

North Carolina State University, The Center for Universal Design. (1997). *What is universal design?* Retrieved March 24, 2004 from, http:// www.design.ncsu.edu:8120/cud/univ_design/princ_overview.htm

Negroponte, N. (1995). *Being digital.* New York: Vintage.

Neuman, W. L. (1997). *Social research methods: Qualitative and quantitative methods.* Toronto, Canada: Allyn & Bacon.

Northrup, P. (2001, March-April). A framework for designing interactivity into Web-based instruction. *Educational Technology,* 31-39.

O'Connor, B. (2000). *E-learning and students with disabilities: From outer edge to leading edge.* Keynote address at NETWorking 2000 Conference, Flexible Learning, Australia. Retrieved May 8, 2003, from http://www .flexiblelearning.net. au/nw2000/main/key04.htm

Opitz, C. (2002). Online course accessibility: A call for responsibility and necessity. *Educational Technology Review, 10*(1). Retrieved May 8, 2003, from http:// www.aace.org/pubs/etr/issue2/optiz-x1.cfm

Owens, C. (1998). The discourse of others: Feminists and postmodernism. In H. Foster (Ed.) *The anti-aesthetic: Essays on postmodern culture* (pp. 65-92). New York: New Press.

Pittinsky, M. S. (2003). *The wired tower: Perspectives on the impact of the Internet on higher education.* Upper Saddle River, NJ: Financial Times Prentice Hall.

Postman, N. (2003). Questioning media. In M. S. Pittinsky (Ed.), *The wired tower: perspectives on the impact of the Internet on higher education* (pp. 181-200). Upper Saddle River, NJ: Financial Times Prentice Hall.

Postman, N. (1993). *The end of education: Redefining the value of school.* New York: Random House.

Postman, N. (1992). *Technopoly: The surrender of culture to technology.* New York: Random House.

Postrel, V. (2003). *The substance of style: How the rise of aesthetic value is remaking commerce, culture & consciousness.* New York: HarperCollins.

The Random house dictionary. (1980). New York: Ballantine.

Robinson, P. (2000). *Within the matrix: A hermeneutic phenomenological investigation of student experiences in a Web-based computer conferencing.* Unpublished doctoral dissertation, University of Maryland.

Scheurich, J. J. (1994). Policy archaeology: A new policy studies methodology. *Journal of Education Policy, 9*(4), 297-316.

Scott, R. A. (1969). *The making of blind men.* New York: Sage.

Searle, J. R. (1995). *The construction of social reality.* New York: The Free Press.

Seelman, K. D. (2001). Science and technology policy: Is disability a missing factor? In G. L. Albrecht, K. D. Seelman, & M. Bury (Eds.), *Handbook of disability studies* (pp. 663-692). Thousand Oaks, CA: Sage.

Shapiro, J. P. (1993). *No pity: People with disabilities forging a new civil rights movement.* New York: Three Rivers.

Spender, D. (1995). *Nattering on the net: Women, power and cyberspace.* Toronto, Ontario, Canada: Garamond.

Spradley, J. P. (1979). *The ethnographic interview.* Fort Worth, TX: Harcourt.

Strathern, P. (2000). *Foucault in 90 Minutes.* Chicago: Ivan R. Dee.

TeleEducation. (n.d.) *The no significant difference phenomenon.* Retrieved June 25, 2003, from http://teleeducation.nb.ca/nosignificantdifference/

tenBroek, J. (1957, July). *Cross of blindness.* An address delivered at the banquet of the annual convention of the National Federation of the Blind, New Orleans, LA. Retrieved September 20, 2002, from http://www.nfb.org/convent/tb1957.htm

The Canadian National Institute for the Blind. (n.d.). *Living with vision loss: A handbook for caregivers.* Retrieved September 4, 2002, from http://www. cnib.ca/eng/publications/pamphlets/1wv1/chapter1.htm

Thompson, M. M. (1998). Distance learners in higher education. In C. C. Gibson (Ed.), *Distance learners in higher education: Institutional responses for quality outcomes* (pp. 9-24). Madison, WI: Atwood.

Twigg, C. A. (2001). *Innovations in online learning: Moving beyond no significant difference.* New York: Center for Academic Transformation. Retrieved September 9, 2002, from http://www.center.rpi.edu/PewSym/Mono4.pdf

Ulster, A .A., & Antle, B. J. (2005). In the darkness there can be light: A family's adaptation to a child's blindness. *Journal of Visual Impairment and Blindness 99*(4), 209-218.

U.S. Department of Education, National Center for Education Statistics. (2001). *Digest of education statistics* (NCES Publication No. 2002-130). Washington, DC: Author.

U.S. Department of Education, National Center for Education Statistics. (1999). *Students with disabilities in postsecondary education: A profile of preparation,participation, and outcomes* (NCES Publication No. 1999-187). Washington, DC: Author.

U.S. Department of Education, National Center for Education Statistics. (1997). *Distance education in higher education institutions* (NCES Publication No. 98-062). Washington, DC: Author.

Usher, R. (1996). Textuality and reflexivity in educational research. In D. Scott & R. Usher (Eds.), *Understanding educational research* (pp. 33-51). New York: Routledge.

van Manen, M. (1997). *Researching lived experience: Human science for an actionsensitive pedagogy.* London, Ontario, Canada: Althouse.

van Manen, M. (2002). *Writing in the dark: Phenomenological studies in interpretive inquiry.* London, Ontario, Canada: Althouse.

Walker, J. (1994). Open Learning: The answer to the government's equity problems? A report of a study on the potential impact of the Open Learning initiative on people with disabilities. *Distance Education, 15*(1), 94-111.

Wileman, R. E. (1980). Exercises ub visual thinking. New York: Hastings House.

Wolf, N. (2002). *The beauty myth: How images of beauty are used against women.* New York: Anchor.

Wolfensberger, W. (1972). *The principle of normalization in human services.* Toronto, Ontario, Canada: National Institute on Mental Retardation.

Printed in the United States
74729LV00001B/22-42

9 781593 115210